"Bassman's book is a guide that everyone can utilize when confronting a problem like fibromyalgia. The right coach will help you to combine inspiration and information, and when you do that, you can expect to achieve exceptional results. *The Feel Good Guide to Fibromyalgia* does it all in a style that is easy to read and use."

—Bernie Siegel, MD, author *Love, Medicine, and Miracles* and *Love, Magic, and Mudpies*

WITHDRAWN   WITHDRAWN

"Bassman has done a fine job of explaining a complex and disabling group of conditions that are underdiagnosed and inadequately treated by mainstream medicine. The solutions she offers are broad-ranging, thorough, user-friendly, individualized, and above all, in the large majority of cases, successful!"

—Hyla Cass, MD, author of *8 Weeks to Vibrant Health: A Woman's Take-Charge Program*

The Feel-Good Guide to Fibromyalgia & Chronic Fatigue Syndrome

A COMPREHENSIVE RESOURCE FOR RECOVERY

LYNETTE BASSMAN, PH.D.

New Harbinger Publications, Inc.

Publisher's Note

Care has been taken to confirm the accuracy of the information presented and to describe generally accepted practices. However, the author, editors, and publisher are not responsible for errors or omissions or for any consequences from application of the information in this book and make no warranty, express or implied, with respect to the contents of the publication.

The author, editors, and publisher have exerted every effort to ensure that any drug selection and dosage set forth in this text are in accordance with current recommendations and practice at the time of publication. However, in view of ongoing research, changes in government regulations, and the constant flow of information relating to drug therapy and drug reactions, the reader is urged to check the package insert for each drug for any change in indications and dosage and for added warnings and precautions. This is particularly important when the recommended agent is a new or infrequently employed drug.

Some drugs and medical devices presented in this publication may have Food and Drug Administration (FDA) clearance for limited use in restricted research settings. It is the responsibility of the health care provider to ascertain the FDA status of each drug or device planned for use in their clinical practice.

Distributed in Canada by Raincoast Books

Copyright © 2007 by Lynette Bassman

New Harbinger Publications, Inc.
5674 Shattuck Avenue
Oakland, CA 94609
www.newharbinger.com

Acquired by Jess O'Brien; Cover design by Amy Shoup;
Edited by Amy Johnson; Text design by Tracy Carlson

Library of Congress Cataloging-in-Publication Data

Bassman, Lynette, 1959-
   The feel-good guide to fibromyalgia and chronic fatigue syndrome : a comprehensive resource for recovery / Lynette Bassman.
      p. cm.
   ISBN 978-1-57224-489-4
   1. Fibromyalgia--Popular works. 2. Chronic fatigue syndrome--Popular works. I. Title.
RC927.3.B39 2007
616.7'42--dc22

                                    2007008087

09 08 07

10 9 8 7 6 5 4 3 2 1   First printing

Contents

Foreword

Every century has certain illnesses that stump physicians. For at least the last half-century fibromyalgia and chronic fatigue have been the bête noir of the medical profession. In the previous century it was neurasthenia, which Florence Nightingale suffered from for many years; chronic fatigue may well be a current version of neurasthenia.

One of the most disturbing aspects of a diagnosis of fibromyalgia or chronic fatigue is that most physicians react as if this means the problem is psychosomatic or all in your head. Nothing could be further from the truth. As this excellent book details, both of these diagnoses are real and can be appropriately treated when they're understood as the body's reactions to multiple stressors: physical, chemical, electromagnetic, and emotional. As Lynette Bassman documents in this book, when stress levels reach a critical point, many body processes begin to break down.

In my decades of clinical work with people in pain, I've found that treatments can be tremendously effective without the use of drugs. As you will see in this thorough, carefully researched book, a wide variety of tools is available to aid you in the recovery process. The good news is that you can feel good again. You have in your hands a wealth of good scientific information to speed you on your road to recovery. Bon voyage!

—C. Norman Shealy, MD, Ph.D.
  President, Holos University Graduate Seminary
  Founding President, American Holistic Medical Association

Acknowledgments

I am grateful to the following people for graciously giving their time to read portions of the manuscript: Larry Bassman, Jem Bluestein, Rosemarie Gladstar, Howard Hurtt, Monika Joshi, Joel Kreisberg, Selena Mitchell, Sue Stone, and Susun Weed. I also appreciate my editors at New Harbinger Publications for their gentle, helpful input, and Josh Johnson and Neal Kennington for research assistance. Thanks also to Bruce Cooperstein and the late Avery Ferentz for putting me on the road to recovery. And I am especially grateful to Jonah Bassman and Larry Bassman for their love, support, and understanding.

Introduction

When you have fibromyalgia (FM) or chronic fatigue syndrome (CFS)—
or think you might—it's not easy to get the health care you need. A lot
of people, doctors included, won't believe you're sick. They may believe
you about nearly any other topic you discuss, but when it comes to
discussing your symptoms, they'll think you don't know what you're
talking about. Even if they accept that FM and CFS exist and your
symptoms are real and debilitating, many people will say that there isn't
much to be done to help. That's not true.

I'm a psychologist and for almost twenty years I've seen people with
FM and CFS and other health problems in my psychotherapy practice.
I know that psychotherapy can help a lot, but I also know that other
healing modalities are needed. Most people don't know much about
these modalities. When a client needs further information, I will often
suggest books they can read. However, when it comes to learning about
the many healing modalities available to help with FM and CFS, there
isn't a book that comprehensively covers the topic. That's why I decided
to write this book.

In addition to my professional experience with these syndromes, I
also have personal experience. Twenty-three years ago I became ill with
what eventually was diagnosed as chronic Epstein-Barr syndrome (an
early name for CFS). Like many people, I went to a conventional MD
for help. He and a rheumatologist ran a lot of tests, considered some
really scary diagnoses, and eventually sent me to see a psychologist.
While psychotherapy was helpful, it didn't make all the symptoms go
away. Luckily, a friend of mine suggested I see his chiropractor, who did
something called applied kinesiology. He described the treatment techniques; they sounded ridiculous. I hesitated, not only because I had no
knowledge of alternative medicine and viewed it as highly suspect, but

also because my health insurance wouldn't cover it and the cost would be difficult for me to manage. But I was desperate, so I went.

That first visit was a revelation. There was no question of whether this chiropractor believed in my illness. Rather than wanting to send me away as my MD had, this doctor was ready to start helping me get better. He had a variety of ways of treating what was going on in my body, and suggested things I could do to help myself, too.

It took a few years, but with nutritional supplements and herbs, dietary changes, bodywork, psychotherapy, and eventually homeopathy and traditional Chinese medicine, I became well. I have been able to stay well by maintaining these dietary changes, exercising regularly, managing stress, avoiding unnecessary toxins, and getting preventive health care.

So I know that people can recover from FM and CFS. I'm grateful my friend pointed me in the right direction and that I was able to try something new and make changes in my life. I hope that this book will point you in the right direction and help inspire you to make any changes you need to recover.

I'll begin by laying the groundwork to help you understand FM and CFS. These first three chapters are very important: not only will they help you get your bearings, they'll also prepare you for making decisions about what healing modalities to use. Chapters 4 through 14 cover a broad range of healing arts that can help with FM and CFS. You can use these chapters as you would a reference book, picking and choosing which ones you want to read based on which methods appeal to you and what you have available in your area or can do as self-care. Or you can read all of the chapters before making any decisions. In addition to the References section at the back of the book, there's also a Resources section that includes helpful Web sites, ways to find different types of practitioners, and other information. Not all of these resources are explicitly referred to elsewhere in the book, so it's a good idea to browse this section to see what's there.

My goal is to give you the information you need, both about what causes your symptoms and about what you can do to feel good again. But I'm not a physician and I can't prescribe treatments. Treatment plans should be tailored to your needs, based on solid diagnostic information. Being an advocate for your own health care is healing in itself; I encourage you to take charge of deciding what is right for you.

One of the lessons to be learned from having FM or CFS is that we need to take very good care of ourselves in order to feel good. By picking up this book, you have begun that process. It is my fondest wish that you will emerge from this illness with the tools to stay well for a lifetime.

CHAPTER 1

Is This Book About You?

What Are Fibromyalgia and Chronic Fatigue Syndrome?

Every day many things must happen in our bodies to maintain healthy, normal functioning. For most people, on most days, these processes go smoothly, without any thought. Sometimes something will go wrong with one of these processes; you might sprain an ankle, impairing your musculoskeletal functioning, or you might develop a stomachache, impairing your digestive functioning. Also, a problem in one system can set off problems in other systems. When this happens it can be hard to figure out what's going wrong.

With fibromyalgia (FM) and chronic fatigue syndrome (CFS), a larger number of basic body processes malfunction—and they don't get better for a long time. The bodies of people with FM and CFS do, however, malfunction in certain characteristic ways; a diagnosis of FM or CFS is based on these characteristic types of dysfunction.

Are CFS and FM the Same Disorder?

CFS and FM are very similar. Some people say they are the same illness. Some people, pointing to specific biological markers that differ between the two groups of patients, say they are different *syndromes*—sets of symptoms that may or may not have a common underlying mechanism. I believe the apparent differences are most likely due to the way the research on these syndromes has been carried out. When you take individuals, each with his or her own unique combination of symptoms, and compare them as groups you lose a lot of specific information. Individuals may seem more alike than they are and groups may seem more different.

Research on CFS grew out of the field of immunology; its early focus was on chronic infections, such as the Epstein-Barr virus, that were often seen in patients with CFS. Research on FM comes from the rheumatology field; its focus was primarily on the pain that people with FM experience. To some degree, the way these two syndromes are defined reflects these roots.

A diagnosis of CFS is based on fatigue and flu-like symptoms, while a diagnosis of FM requires a certain number of tender points on specific parts of your body. But most people with FM will tell you that they have fatigue and most people with CFS will tell you that they ache all over. Also, individual doctors may diagnose you with one or the other as a result of knowing more about that particular syndrome and being sensitized through their own training to focus on certain symptoms that fit their understanding of the illness.

Because FM often follows a physical trauma, such as an automobile accident, and CFS often follows an illness, such as mononucleosis or a severe flu, it may be that the terms FM and CFS are actually names for two subgroups of the same syndrome, triggered differently.

So, although it's not clear yet whether these two syndromes are really the same illness, they have so many elements in common that, until new information comes to light that clearly differentiates between them, there is more reason to assume they're the same than to assume they're different.

Do You Have One of These Syndromes?

A diagnosis of FM or CFS is made by comparing your symptoms to a list of symptoms characteristic of the illness. The diagnostic criteria for both FM and CFS are works in progress; they've been revised in the light of new information and will probably be revised again. Diagnosing a syndrome is different than diagnosing a disease, the criteria for which might include not just a list of symptoms but also a blood test or some other marker that distinguishes between those with the disease and those without it. So far, for FM and CFS there's no distinguishing marker. Unfortunately, some people make the mistake of thinking this means these illnesses aren't real.

With any set of diagnostic criteria, there are typically people who meet all of the criteria, people who meet the minimum number of criteria, and some who fall just short of the criteria. On the other hand, there are many, many symptoms that don't appear in the criteria because whoever wrote the criteria didn't deem these symptoms representative of enough of the people with the illnesses. So, although diagnostic criteria are helpful, they shouldn't be regarded as any kind of ultimate truth.

If you don't meet the full criteria for FM or for CFS, but you're experiencing a lot of similar types of dysfunction, you may still find the information in this book helpful to you.

Diagnosis Step One: Ruling out Other Disorders

There are a variety of disorders that can masquerade as FM or CFS but require different treatment. FM and CFS can only be diagnosed when these other disorders have been ruled out. However, some people do have both one of these other illnesses and FM or CFS. Your MD will know what tests to run to rule these other disorders out:

autoimmune disease	mitochondrial disease
cancer	multiple sclerosis
early Parkinson's disease	myofascial pain syndrome
eating disorders	narcolepsy and other sleep disorders
generalized osteoarthritis	obesity
hepatitis	osteomalacia
hormonal disorders	polymyalgia rheumatica
hypothyroidism	subacute infections
lupus	

Diagnosis Step Two: Checking the Diagnostic Criteria

If, with the help of a health care professional, you've ruled out the above diagnoses, check the following two sets of criteria to see if your symptoms fit either diagnosis.

The American College of Rheumatology Criteria for Fibromyalgia (Wolfe et al. 1990)

- Pain must be present in eleven of eighteen specific points on the body when moderate pressure is applied. Pictures showing the locations of these points can be found on many FM Web sites. An examination of these tender points must be carefully carried out by a health professional who has training in the proper procedure.

- The pain must be in all four quadrants of the body, plus the cervical spine, anterior chest, thoracic spine, or lower back.

- The pain must have been present for at least three months.

CDC Revised Criteria for Chronic Fatigue Syndrome (Fukuda et al. 1994)

- Severe, unexplained, persistent chronic fatigue.

- Four or more of the following symptoms for six or more months, not predating the fatigue: substantial impairment in short-term memory or concentration; sore throat; tender lymph nodes; muscle pain; multijoint pain without swelling or redness; headaches of a new type, pattern, or severity; unrefreshing sleep; and postexertional malaise lasting more than twenty-four hours.

Diagnosis Step Three: Identifying Additional Symptoms

The following are some additional symptoms and co-occurring conditions that many people with FM and CFS experience (bear in mind that these can be symptoms of many other health conditions as well):

abdominal pain	irregular heartbeat
alcohol intolerance	irritable bowel, colitis
anxiety and panic attacks	irritability
bloating	jaw pain (TMJ)
brain fog	low-grade fever
chronic cough	memory difficulties
depression	mitral valve prolapse
diarrhea	nausea
dizziness	neurally mediated hypotension and fainting
dry eyes or mouth	night sweats
dysmenorrhea	osteoporosis
earaches	sensitivity to loud noises, bright lights, odors, drugs, and chemicals
endometriosis	shortness of breath
esophageal dysmotility	skin problems
headache (migraine and other types)	sleep disturbance
interstitial cystitis	tingling sensations

Is It All in Your Head?

Because depression and anxiety are common in people with FM and CFS, many uninformed people claim these illnesses don't really exist, that they're all in your head. However, anxiety and depression appear to be just two of the many symptoms of these illnesses and there's no indication that either is the cause of the other symptoms. Also, it's well established that the bodies of people with FM or CFS demonstrate very real, physical differences compared with healthy bodies.

You may have encountered health care providers who imply that you're somehow fabricating your symptoms or trying to make them seem worse than they are. One survey of doctors found that a full half didn't "believe in" FM and CFS (Thomas and Smith 2005). The mainstream medical literature is now so full of articles about the very real physical changes that occur in FM and CFS that there's really no reason for any doctor to be unaware of these syndromes and their medical bases.

What Causes FM and CFS?

To get a more complete answer to the question of what causes FM and CFS, you need to know the meanings of two words: *allopathic* and *holistic*. In allopathic, or conventional, medicine, as practiced by nearly all physicians in the U.S. for the last hundred years, it's believed that there's a single cause for each problem, e.g., a lesion, deficiency, infection, injury, etc. Treatment aims to fight that cause. From a holistic point of view, there are multiple causes for multiple symptoms; the body is a system and everything affects everything else; causes can be subtle. Treatment usually works in harmony with the body's self-healing mechanisms.

Allopathic Versus Holistic Views of FM and CFS

Although researchers agree that FM is a disorder of central processing with neuroendocrine/neurotransmitter dysregulation, from the allopathic point of view, there's no known cause of either FM or CFS. But this is a result of approaching the question with the idea that a single cause must be found for everybody who has the illness. From a holistic point of view, the cause of the illness is unique to each individual and can be determined by a number of methods.

Ever since allopathic medicine came on the scene there has been conflict between these two ways of looking at human health. In recent years, proponents of the two points of view have begun dialogues with each other, and many allopathic physicians have started to incorporate holistic treatments into their practice. Interestingly, it appears that chronic illnesses like CFS and FM have been a catalyst for this change. As a result, the dividing line between allopathic treatment and holistic treatments has blurred, and the field of integrative medicine has emerged. This is a very fortunate development—it means that many people now have access to treatments that were previously either unavailable or frowned upon by their doctors and others.

There is a negative side to this development, too, however. Applying an allopathic view to treatments that arise from a holistic tradition can weaken these treatments. For example, acupuncture, the main tool of traditional Chinese medicine, is much more accepted today than in the past and is now being practiced by many MDs; as a result, it's now more readily available. But many of the programs that train physicians to use acupuncture take it out of context. It's often used for symptomatic relief, or to counter the effects of some pathogen or lesion. Although this can be effective, it's not as effective as using acupuncture in the context of the holistic conceptualization of the body, where needling and other approaches are used to restore the normal flow of chi—or life energy—throughout the body, which in turn improves the health of the whole person in a more lasting way. Many physicians who practice acupuncture will tell you that they do not believe that there is such a thing as chi—and yet this concept is central to the healing art they're practicing.

Causes of FM and CFS from a Holistic Point of View

From a holistic point of view, it appears that usually more than one of the following plays a role in causing FM and CFS:

Emotional Stress and Other Kinds of Stress

When we hear the word "stress," we typically think of emotional stress. Emotional stress is a major factor in FM and CFS. However, stress can be anything that takes your body out of balance. So, for example, if you work in a very cold or hot environment, your body must work hard to maintain a normal body temperature. This is *thermal stress*. If you wear high-heeled shoes, your usual balance mechanisms can't be used as effectively and your body must struggle to find other ways to keep from falling. This is *mechanical stress*.

When faced with just a few minor stressors, your body can use its natural healing abilities to restore equilibrium. However, a very large stressor—or many stressors—can overtax the ability of your body to heal itself and symptoms will result. Sometimes, the ways that your body adapts to stressors can become problems in and of themselves; for example, when your body isn't getting enough dietary calcium (*nutritional stress*) it will use the calcium in your bones to compensate; weak bones may then result.

The *diathesis stress* model suggests that although some people may have a predisposition or a vulnerability to a certain illness—through defects in metabolism, detoxification, neuroendocrine functioning, and other body processes—they may not get symptoms of the illness unless triggers activate that potential.

Pathogens and Impaired Immune Response

Some people become ill with CFS (more so than those with FM) following an illness. If the immune system is compromised, it can't fight off infection as well as normally and an infection can become chronic.

Physical Trauma

Many people with FM (more so than those with CFS) report that their symptoms began following a physical trauma, often an automobile accident. This seems to set off a series of events in the body that lead to widespread pain and other symptoms.

Psychological Styles and Childhood History

FM and CFS patients show a higher than normal amount of childhood trauma. The group also seems to contain a higher than average number of people with a strongly goal-oriented approach to life.

Poor Nutrition

The foods that most of us eat don't support healthy bodies. They are too processed, grown in soil that lacks nutrients, and shipped long distances, so that they are rarely eaten when fresh. Typically we then doctor them with harmful additives: preservatives, too much salt, the wrong fats, and flavor-enhancing chemicals.

Toxic Exposures

In addition to the toxins in the foods we eat, we also consume hundreds of poisons every day in our water and our air. After a critical amount, our bodies can no longer cope with these poisons and start to react.

Genetics

Family members of patients with FM and CFS display a higher than average frequency of the syndromes as well as conditions related to them, including irritable bowel syndrome, migraine headaches, and mood disorders. It's possible that rather than inheriting a specific FM or CFS gene, what's actually inherited is a factor that predisposes individuals to acquiring a chronic multisystem illness—such as an environmental sensitivity, a different way of processing nutrients, a tendency toward a certain kind of personality, or a shortage of a certain brain chemical, particularly those involved in the stress response. (See the Resources section for information about the CFS Computational Challenge, a series of studies about the genetic basis of CFS.)

Multiple Causes, Multiple Effects

Some people say that more than anything else, FM and CFS are illnesses caused by our modern lifestyle. We eat poorly, don't relax enough, and are exposed every day to hundreds of toxins and an overload of information. Although some people appear to escape the ill effects of this, those with FM or CFS—or heart disease, asthma, diabetes, etc.—have the dubious distinction of having bodies that react to this unhealthy lifestyle. Consider this a wake-up call—we have the chance to make changes before it's too late. This book aims to help you understand both what's going wrong with your body and the different options you have to make these changes.

Chapter 2

Why Do You Feel So Sick?

FM and CFS are syndromes that have complex sets of symptoms, often with one problem triggering a cascading series of additional symptoms. This can be both confusing and overwhelming. However, although the functioning of the body may be complex, it's not beyond understanding.

This chapter will review the main systems of the body, what they do when they work as they should, and the ways that they tend to malfunction in people with FM and CFS. You will notice that there are more systems covered here than the standard organ systems you may have learned about in school; this is reflective of a more holistic view of health that incorporates mind, body, and spirit. The fourteen elements of health are: respiration and oxygenation, nutrition, digestion and metabolism, nerve transmission, immune response, repair of free radical damage, circulation, detoxification, hormonal balance, structural alignment and balance, sleep and restoration, emotional response, spiritual wellness, and the balance of subtle energies.

Each of these fourteen elements could be—and often is—the focus of entire graduate level courses and textbooks, so the coverage here will necessarily be somewhat superficial. My goal is to give you the information you need in language that's easy to absorb, so that you have the terminology you need to talk to your health care providers or do further research. I will also provide you with guidelines for determining whether a given system is problematic for you. If you know what's causing your symptoms, it's easier to figure out what kinds of treatments are appropriate.

Respiration and Oxygenation

Oxygen is critical to your health. Without oxygen you can survive only a few minutes, whereas without food and water you can survive much longer. Respiration actually involves two related processes: breathing or ventilation, and blood and cell oxygenation.

Ventilation or Breathing

The first part of the respiration process is *ventilation* or breathing. When you breathe, you take in oxygen and expel carbon dioxide. This exchange happens in small air sacs in the lungs called *alveoli*. Oxygen is moved from alveoli into the blood, while carbon dioxide is moved out of the blood through capillaries. Ventilation isn't usually a problem for people with FM or CFS.

Blood and Cell Oxygenation

In the second phase of respiration, *cell respiration*, cells are provided with energy in the form of *adenosine triphosphate* (ATP) through a series of chemical reactions between the oxygen and the carbohydrates you eat. (Carbon dioxide is a byproduct of this process.) When cells don't get enough oxygen, the result can be pain, fatigue, muscle weakness, low energy, heart and brain dysfunction, shortness of breath, pallor, slow healing, or other symptoms. This can be diagnosed through a *blood gas analysis*, a test that measures the levels of oxygen and carbon dioxide in your blood, or through a blood test for *hemoglobin*, the protein in your blood that carries oxygen and carbon dioxide. Abnormal hemoglobin levels are fairly common in people with FM and CFS.

Blood and cell oxygenation may be hindered by a hereditary or acquired tendency for blood to coagulate, or thicken. This tendency is activated when the body encounters an infection, which is why it is called *immune system activation of coagulation* (ISAC) (Berg et al. 1999). This increased thickness then makes the blood less able to carry oxygen to cells. Because this is seen more frequently in people with FM and CFS and other chronic illnesses than in the general population, it's hypothesized that this may be an important factor in these syndromes.

Cell respiration requires coenzyme Q_{10} (Co Q 10), iron, copper, B_1, B_2, B_3, B_5, manganese, lipoic acid, biotin, magnesium (Schmitt 2005), vitamins E and K, and nicotinamide adenine dinucleotide (Kidd 2005). A lack of these nutrients will interfere with production of ATP. According to Schmitt (2005), *heavy metal toxicity*—a buildup of substances such as mercury and lead in the tissues of the body—can also interfere with this process. Besides leading to lower ATP supplies, both heavy metal toxicity and immune responses lead to buildups of lactic acid, pyruvic acid, and other organic acids involved in cell respiration. These can be measured by urine organic acid profiles (Schmitt 2005).

Another factor that can interfere with the production of ATP is excess amounts of *tartaric acid*, a byproduct of yeast fermentation. Excess tartaric acid will block the production of *malic acid*, an intermediary in cell respiration and one of the regulators of blood sugar (Abraham and Flechas 1992); low blood sugar is quite common among people with FM and CFS. Excess tartaric acid may also be a cause of the pain and weakness experienced by people with FM and CFS (St. Amand and Marek 2003).

Mitochondria are the small structures in your cells that make ATP, so if your mitochondria aren't working well, you may develop a variety of symptoms as a result. There appears to be a tendency in people with FM and CFS for inherited dysfunction of the mitochondria (Kaushik et al. 2005). In addition, many other processes involved in the symptoms of FM and CFS also interfere with the mitochondria. Chronic infection, as commonly seen in people with FM and CFS, damages the mitochondria, as do *free radicals*—unstable molecules created by the normal metabolic processes of your body. If the integrity of the membranes of the mitochondria is compromised, the balance of *electrolytes*—minerals that carry an electrical charge and are important for fluid balance and muscle activity among other functions—may be disturbed.

Majid Ali (2003) hypothesizes that one cause of the weakness, fatigue, and brain fog seen in FM and CFS is that due to problems with the availability and functioning of mitochondrial enzymes, the body produces ATP by an additional pathway, called *fermentation*. Fermentation doesn't require oxygen, but produces energy with much less efficiency than does the oxygen-based respiration. Ali believes that the accuracy of his *RTF hypothesis*—RTF stands for "respiration to fermentation"—can be verified by tests for certain organic acids excreted in urine. Greatly elevated levels of these substances have been found in people with FM and CFS.

Nutrition

Poor nutrition affects many aspects of our functioning. Many nutritional deficiencies can be measured through blood or urine tests; some labs even specialize in nutritional profiles. However, because these tests can be very expensive and variable over time, some basic signs of nutritional deficiency to look for are: failure to maintain a healthy weight; pale skin; changes in fingernails, skin, or hair; bleeding gums; dark circles under the eyes; heart disease; changes in the color or quantity of urine; goiter; poor circulation; and constipation or diarrhea. This list could actually go on for many pages—and would include most of the symptoms of FM and CFS.

Nutritional Deficiencies Seen in FM and CFS

The following is a brief sampling of nutrition issues commonly seen in people with CFS and FM (other than toxicity or food allergies, which are covered in separate sections):

Amino Acid Deficiencies/Excesses

One researcher divides people with FM and CFS into six different groups, based on different specific distributions (depletion or excess) of thirteen *amino acids*—building blocks of protein. These distribution patterns differ from those found in people without FM or CFS. It is unclear, though, whether amino acid problems are a cause of the syndromes or a result (Dunstan et al. 2000).

Regland et al. (1997) found high levels of the amino acid *homocysteine* in people with FM and CFS, and suggests that this may be partly due to low cerebrospinal fluid levels of vitamin B_{12}. High homocysteine levels have been found to be correlated with fatigue (Regland et al. 1997).

Magnesium Deficiency

Many factors can deplete magnesium, and without sufficient magnesium, pain may be increased (Mauskop et al. 1996). Eisinger et al. (1994) found that people with FM and CFS have suboptimal proportions of calcium and magnesium, which work synergistically and need to be kept in balance for good health. Calcium-magnesium imbalances may be due to malabsorption or inadequate dietary intake of these minerals or vitamin D, which is needed for their utilization.

Vitamin D Deficiency

In addition to being involved in bone formation, vitamin D is crucial for many aspects of immune system functioning (Cantorna et al. 2004) and for pain regulation (Plotnikoff and Quigley 2003); therefore, a deficiency could be a causative factor in FM and CFS. Holick and Jenkins (2005) and others believe that a deficiency of this vitamin is more common than previously thought.

Additional Nutritional Deficiencies

Other nutritional deficiencies commonly seen in people with FM and CFS include deficiencies in malic acid, B vitamins, manganese, electrolytes, trace minerals, vitamin C and other antioxidants, and essential fatty acids (Werbach 2000). Each of these nutrients performs multiple important functions; if you're deficient in any of them, you may be at risk for a variety of health problems.

Digestion and Metabolism

Even if you eat the ideal diet for your body, problems in the absorption or utilization of nutrients can cause health problems such as those seen in FM and CFS.

Your digestive tract is basically a long muscular tube that excretes digestive juices at various points along its length. The tube's muscles move in waves to keep things moving along; this movement is called *peristalsis*. The following are the steps in the process of digestion:

1. First, in your mouth, chewing breaks food down into more manageable pieces. Additionally, food is mixed with saliva, which both lubricates it for smooth passage and contains enzymes that begin the process of starch digestion.

2. Next, after you swallow, food passes along the esophagus, through a valve, and into the stomach, where it may stay for as long as a few hours. There, it is mixed with stomach acid and enzymes that begin to digest any protein.

3. From the stomach, the now partially digested food passes into the small intestine, where it is mixed with more digestive juices from the pancreas, liver, and intestine, which neutralize its acidity and contain enzymes that further break down the proteins, fats, and carbohydrates. Bile, a product of the liver that emulsifies fats to hasten their digestion, is also introduced.

4. Nutrients then pass through *mucosa*—the permeable walls of the small intestine—and into the bloodstream, whereupon they are then filtered through the liver before being transported to other locations in the body.

5. Waste material—and any dead cells that the digestive tract has shed—is moved into the large intestine, or colon. In the colon, water is absorbed and any remaining usable food is broken down, or fermented, by the bacteria that live there. The remaining material is then stored in the rectum until it is expelled during a bowel movement.

Regulation of Digestion

The process of digestion is regulated in two different ways: through chemicals that control the release of the various juices and through nerve action. Brain chemicals trigger the digestive process to either activate or slow down. For example, when you see and smell something good to eat, unconscious processes in the brain and spinal cord trigger salivation. The same chemical messengers that are found in the brain are also found in the *enteric nervous system*, the processing center located in the gut. However, this complex network of nerves is triggered by the mechanical force of food along the walls of the tract; this force stretches the walls and causes the process to speed up or slow down. The enteric and the central nervous systems normally work cooperatively to manage the connections between digestion and other body functions.

Irritable Bowel and Related Syndromes

If the various parts of the digestive system aren't cooperating properly, the result may be irritable bowel syndrome (IBS), which is quite common in people with FM and CFS. It appears IBS is caused not by any actual physical lesion, but by problems in the communication of nerves between the brain, spinal cord, and intestinal tract. This may be part of the larger pattern of systemic oversensitivity common in CFS and FM, and seen in excessive reactions of the nervous system to touch, light, temperature, or sound. The symptoms of IBS are alternating diarrhea and constipation, gas, painful spasms, and bloating.

Incomplete digestion of *lactose*—the sugar in milk—and *fructose*—a sugar naturally found in many fruits and a sweetener used in many processed foods—is sometimes associated with IBS. Ringel, Sperber, and Drossman (2001) speculate that IBS may follow an inflammation due to a bacterial infection of the bowel. It is also believed that IBS can be caused by food allergies (Zar, Benson, and Kumar 2005).

Our intestines are host to a number of organisms that help with the work of digestion. Sometimes, due to a decrease in the stomach acids or digestive enzymes that normally keep these organisms in proper balance, one or more of these organisms will proliferate. It has been proposed that excess amounts of these organisms may cause IBS and Crohn's disease, a related problem (Pimentel, Chow, and Lin 2000). *Dysbiosis* refers to the overgrowth of these organisms, which include yeasts like *Candida albicans*, parasites like *Giardia lamblia*, and bacteria like *salmonella*. Crook (1999) has developed both a questionnaire-type test and a saliva test that may help to determine if yeast overgrowth is a problem for you.

One theory about IBS and related inflammatory bowel diseases is that they're caused by the immune system attacking the beneficial bacteria normally found in the intestine; this attack includes increasing white blood cells, which then causes inflammation. Over time, this creates harmful byproducts that damage the walls of the intestine (Elson et al. 2003).

Leaky Gut Syndrome and Food Sensitivities

A common dysfunction in the digestive systems of people with FM and CFS is *leaky gut syndrome*. According to Leo Galland (1998), a leading expert in the field, when the walls of the intestines are inflamed their permeability is affected. Increased gut permeability may also be due to parasites, poor diet, smoking, alcohol, nonsteroidal anti-inflammatory drugs, and antibiotics.

If the gut is too permeable, molecules of food can get into the bloodstream before they have been sufficiently broken down. This can cause adverse reactions to food—commonly referred to as food sensitivities or intolerances—because the body sees these particles as invading organisms and develops antibodies to them. In the process of attacking these partially digested food particles, antibodies sometimes attack the body's tissues as well, leading to a host of other symptoms (Cutler 2003). This process is one form of autoimmune disease.

If the efficiency of the gut's internal immune processes is lowered, it may lead to similar, associated sensitivities to the bacteria, viruses, and yeasts normally present. In addition, some toxic material may get through the barrier that's supposed to protect the rest of the body from the normal byproducts of digestion. This then places a burden on the liver, making it less able to carry out its normal functions. If the liver can't keep up, your body may then accumulate toxins, creating a further need for an immune response, which can then further tax your liver's ability to protect you—leaving you vulnerable to infections the body would normally fight off with ease.

Food sensitivities are very common in people with FM and CFS, affecting as many as 84 percent, according to one study (Thiel 1998). But if you have food sensitivities, you may not know it. Sometimes it's difficult to identify the associations between particular foods and the symptoms that result, due to a considerable time lag between consumption of food and onset of symptoms. Also, if you're sensitive to foods that you consume often, you may never have times when you're symptom-free, making it difficult to pinpoint what causes the symptoms. And because most of us are accustomed to thinking of allergies as producing certain characteristic symptoms—skin rashes, difficulties in breathing, and upper respiratory symptoms—we may not consider food sensitivities as likely culprits for symptoms such as fatigue, headaches, brain fog, and joint pain (Farah et al. 1985).

One way to determine if you're experiencing food sensitivities is to eliminate one food from your diet at a time and track any changes in your symptoms that may result (see the Resources section for a Web site that can assist in this process). You can also use antigen testing, applied kinesiology muscle testing (see chapter 8), or stool, urine, pulse, or breath tests to determine if a specific food is causing a problem. In some cases, since any food can trigger a sensitivity in a person whose gut is overly permeable, a supervised fast may be the best way to test for food intolerances until there has been sufficient healing.

Reflux

Another problem with the digestive process occurs when the valve between the esophagus and stomach doesn't do its job properly, allowing food to back up. This is called *gastroesophageal reflux* and causes heartburn, irritation, and sometimes nausea. A similar problem sometimes happens with the ileocecal valve, which controls the movement of food from the small intestine to the large intestine. When this valve doesn't function properly, food can pass too quickly into the large intestine and waste material can back up into the small intestine.

Malabsorption of Nutrients

Some people with FM and CFS are malnourished due to a malabsorption of nutrients from food. When inflammation damages carrier proteins, the vitamins and minerals that normally pass through the wall of the gut via these proteins may no longer be absorbed. This can result in nutritional deficiencies that then cause additional symptoms that can in turn weaken your body's ability to keep you well.

Nerve Transmission

Because the nervous system is central to our functioning, when it malfunctions there are far-reaching effects on the body. Most scientists who study FM and CFS believe the nervous system is at the core of these syndromes.

There are two parts to the nervous system: the *central nervous system* (CNS)—the brain and spinal cord—and the *peripheral nervous system* (PNS)—the rest of the nerves in the body. The CNS processes and distributes information and is the seat of consciousness and reflexes. The PNS collects sensory information and distributes instructions to organs and muscles.

The PNS is composed of the *autonomic nervous system*, which is primarily involuntary, and the *somatic*, or *sensory nervous system*. The autonomic nervous system has three parts:

- The *enteric nervous system*, which is involved in the functioning of your gastrointestinal tract, gall bladder, and pancreas.

- The *sympathetic branch*, which prepares you for quick responses to challenges, often referred to as the fight-or-flight response.

- The *parasympathetic branch*, which is involved in calming your body—e.g., lowering your heart rate or blood pressure—and supporting the digestion of food.

The sympathetic and the parasympathetic branches have opposite actions. Normally they're in balance. Sometimes, however, they get out of balance and one or the other dominates. This is known as *dysautonomia* and is very common in people with FM and CFS.

Low Blood Pressure

One of the prime signs of dysautonomia frequently seen in people with FM and CFS is *neurally mediated hypotension* (NMH)—low blood pressure resulting from a faulty feedback loop between the brain and the heart, although neither one of these organs may have any gross pathology (Martinez-Lavin 2004). Generally, people with NMH have lower blood pressure when they stand up, which sometimes leads to fainting. (Normally blood pressure rises when a person stands up to compensate for the postural change.) NMH can be measured through the use of a *tilt table test*, where a person lies on a special table and blood pressure is taken repeatedly as the table is gradually tilted to a vertical position. You may be able to informally assess whether you have NMH by noticing whether you often feel as if you're going to pass out when you stand up quickly.

Neurotransmitters

The parts of the nervous system use *neurotransmitters*—chemical messengers that transmit signals that travel from one neuron to the next—to communicate with each other. There are a number of different neurotransmitters; each has its own role.

People with FM and CFS display some differences in the levels and functioning of neurotransmitters. For example, in people with FM there's a tendency toward lower levels of the neurotransmitter *serotonin*, and higher levels in people with CFS (Juhl 1998). Among other things, serotonin regulates pain signals coming into the brain (Badawy et al. 2005). Research has also suggested people with FM have high levels of the neurotransmitter *norepinephrine* (Martinez-Lavin 2004), as well as probable alterations in the efficiency of the neurotransmitter *dopamine* in both people with FM and those with CFS. Buskila and Neumann (2005) believe that people with FM and CFS may have an inherited tendency for differences in their serotonin and dopamine systems.

Some Differences Found in People with FM and CFS

The *cerebrospinal fluid* of people with FM and CFS appears to contain some specific nervous system and immune system proteins that aren't present in the cerebrospinal fluid of people without these syndromes. (Cerebrospinal fluid acts as a shock absorber for the brain, compensating for any changes in the volume of the brain tissue.) The implications of this aren't yet clear, but these twenty proteins may eventually serve as a way to definitively diagnose these syndromes; undoubtedly they will help us understand the underlying mechanisms of the syndromes, which may by itself help us identify effective treatments (Baraniuk et al. 2005).

Another recent finding is that people with CFS have reduced gray matter in their brains (de Lange et al. 2005). This appears to be related to reduced levels of physical activity, but the exact nature of this relationship needs further exploration.

Central Sensitivity Syndromes

There are a number of findings related to hypersensitivity of the nervous systems of people with FM or CFS, which Muhammad Yunus (2001) has called *central sensitivity syndromes* (CSS). Yunus states that there are a number of conditions associated with CSS, including FM and CFS, irritable bowel syndrome, restless leg syndrome, myofascial pain, and others. According to Yunus, people with CSS show signs of a hypersensitivity to stimuli—e.g., touch, light, odors, and temperature—that stems from dysfunction in the CNS. Here are just some of the findings that support the idea of CSS:

- Kramis, Roberts, and Gillette (1996) have found that this central nervous system hypersensitivity can cause pain for which no pathology can be found at the site of the pain. The pathways involved in the sensation of this pain are different from those that mediate pain caused by a wound. This so-called *nonnociceptive* pain originates instead in the *hypothalamic-pituitary-adrenal axis* (HPA axis), the body's stress response system.

- Russell (1998) has found higher levels of *substance P*—a neurotransmitter involved in the communication of pain, touch, and temperature from the body to the brain—in people with FM and, to a lesser degree, in people with CFS. It's believed that this is one of the causes of the increased pain sensitivity seen in these syndromes.

- Staud (2004) suggests that there may be changes in both nerve endings and the rest of the nervous system that may cause normally innocuous stimuli to be experienced as pain and quickly overwhelm the person.

- Nijs, Van de Velde, and De Meirleir (2005) suggest that changes in the way pain is sensed may be due to excess nitric oxide in the body caused by various infectious agents, such as mycoplasma or the Coxsackie B virus.

- Laske et al. (2006) found that *brain-derived neurotrophic factor* (BDNF)—a protein involved in pain sensation—is higher in people with FM than healthy controls, which may explain increased pain sensitivity.

- Gracely et al. (2002) found that pain centers in the brains of people with FM and CFS are activated by much lower levels of pressure than for people without these syndromes. Imaging studies have also found increased blood flow in the *anterior cingulate*—the area of the brain that processes the unpleasantness of pain.

Additional Neurological Findings

One way to study the functioning of the different parts of the brain is to observe the levels of blood flowing to them. Low levels of blood flow were found in the areas of the brains of people with FM and CFS that process senses other than the sense of smell (Kwiatek et al. 2000); movement regulation, memory, and concentration (Mountz et al. 1995); fatigue (Cleare et al. 2005); and stress and emotional responses (Goldstein 1993). There is also less usage of glucose by the brain, which might explain symptoms such as brain fog.

It's not yet clear whether these findings represent causes of FM and CFS symptoms or results of these symptoms.

Immune Response

We live with a large number of organisms, both inside and outside our bodies. This may sound unappealing, but it's a fact of life and in most people doesn't cause a problem. Organisms that are from outside our bodies may enter our bodies through our nose, eyes, mouth, skin, digestive tract, or genitals. Provided there aren't too many of them, they aren't particularly powerful, and the body's defenses are adequate to the task of fighting them off, this works out fine.

How the Immune System Works

The first and most basic way our immune system protects us from invading organisms is with physical barriers to prevent pathogens from getting in. These include the skin and the mucous membranes that line the nose, mouth, and gut. For example, if an irritant arrives in your nose your body will try to expel it by sneezing. If these barriers fail to keep out a harmful organism, a complex interaction of defense mechanisms then takes over. *White blood cells* are a major player in this process.

White blood cells are made in the bone marrow and carried by the circulatory system to wherever they are needed. Roughly half of them migrate to your thymus gland and eventually become helper T, killer T, memory T, or suppressor T cells. The remaining half become macrophages, natural killer (NK) cells, or B cells (Collinge 1993).

The following is a brief summary of the roles played by each of these immune system components:

Helper T cells serve to activate the immune system. After receiving signals from other cells that there is a problem, they release *cytokines*—chemical messengers—to get things going.

Suppressor T cells participate in informing other immune cells when their mission is accomplished.

Killer T cells are one of the various cells that carry the message from helper T cells that a response is needed and what kind; they also start to attack the offending organism.

Macrophages engulf and digest waste of various kinds all around the body. Because they are constantly scanning, they can be the first to recognize the presence of a pathogen. When they do, they send a message to helper T cells, describing the pathogen that has been found.

Natural killer cells function independently and specialize in identifying and disarming cancer cells and cells infected by viruses. They attack in much the same way as killer T cells and, in fact, do the same work as killer T cells but without depending on T cells—which makes them able to fill in for killer T cells when necessary.

B cells function differently from other immune cells. By circulating in the bloodstream and *lymphatic fluid* rather than working directly at the site of a pathogen invasion they exert a more general influence on the body. (Lymphatic fluid is a clear liquid that circulates throughout the body in special vessels that parallel the blood circulatory vessels. These vessels meet at lymph nodes, which serve as staging areas for several types of immune cells—as do the spleen, lymphatic tissue in the tonsils and adenoids, the appendix, and immune tissue in the small intestine.) When B cells get the message that an invasion has occurred, they begin to produce antibodies, called *immunoglobulin* (Ig). Ig attaches itself to a virus and deactivates it until a macrophage can digest it and take it away. When this happens, the antibody is taken as well. B cells produce antibodies for every pathogen that you're exposed to, storing the memory of how to make it, so that in the event that you are reexposed to the same pathogen the proper antibody can quickly be made and deployed. Providing all goes well, B cells produce an amount of Ig that's just right for the size of the invading pathogen.

Immune Dysfunction in FM and CFS

In people with FM and CFS, problems with the immune system are nearly universal. There are two general categories of these problems: immune systems that are underactive, failing to mount responses sufficient to handle threats facing the body, and immune systems that are overactive, responding excessively to circumstances.

In underactive immune systems there isn't a good match between the threat and the response to the threat. This appears to be what happens when people with FM or CFS have an ongoing infection that seems to take forever to heal. The immune response is not sufficient to handle the threat.

When an immune system is overactive it may mount a defense against the body's own tissues, harming or destroying them—as is the case with multiple sclerosis and rheumatoid arthritis, both autoimmune disorders. FM and CFS aren't considered autoimmune disorders but some studies have found similar autoimmune processes active in people with CFS (Vernon and Reeves 2005). The multiple food sensitivities and allergies seen in FM and CFS are also signs of overactive immune systems—inadequately digested food components are attacked as if they are offending organisms. Wheatland (2005) proposes autoimmune reactions to the body's neurotransmitter *ACTH* as the causative factor in the HPA axis problems that are so central to FM and CFS (see section on hormonal balance, this chapter).

With FM and CFS, we see elements of both underactive and overactive immune function (Collinge 1993). In people with FM or CFS there tend to be larger numbers of T cells and extremely elevated levels of cytokines—particularly when the illness is further developed (Wallace et al. 2001). There are also immunoglobulin deficiencies and irregularities of *perforin*, a chemical weapon that T cells use against bacteria (Maher, Klimas, and Fletcher 2005). Functional deficiencies of natural killer (NK) cells are seen even when there may be a sufficient or even an excessive number of NK cells (Robertson et al. 2005). It has been proposed that the tendency for low NK cell activity is inherited (Kaushik et al. 2005). It should be noted, though, that some research found no significant abnormalities in NK cell levels in people with FM or CFS (Landis et al. 2004).

Inflammatory Processes

Inflammation is part of the body's immune response and a necessary component of proper functioning. Typically inflammation isn't directly associated with FM and CFS. With FM and CFS there's no inflammation at the site of the pain as there can be with rheumatoid arthritis and repetitive stress injuries; since the pain is initiated in the CNS, there's little or no pathology at the site of the pain. However, inflammation does play a role in FM and CFS. People with CFS have been found to have higher than normal levels of C-reactive protein, beta 2-microglobulin, and neopterin, all indicators of inflammation (Buchwald et al. 1997), as well as cytokines, whose main job is to activate immune response through inflammation (Wallace et al. 2001). One recent study (Lucas et al. 2006) found increased numbers of activated *mast cells*—immune system components in the skin that trigger inflammatory and neurosensitizing processes—in the skin of people with FM and CFS in response to hormone release. People with FM and CFS have also responded well to replacement of a naturally occurring anti-inflammatory substance that some people lack due to a genetic flaw (Blanco et al. 2005). Additionally, as we have seen, chronic inflammation of the digestive tract is common in people with FM and CFS.

Chronic Immune System Activation

Patients with FM and CFS consistently display chronically activated immune systems (Bates et al. 1995). Chronic activation of the immune system can produce a range of side effects. Cytokines, messengers of the immune system's helper T cells, generate waste products that can cross the blood-brain barrier and that can damage brain tissue if they build up (Szelenyi 2001). Because some of the parts of the brain they damage are involved in immune function, a vicious cycle is created, making it extremely difficult to heal. Chronic immune system activation can also interrupt neurotransmitters that affect blood pressure, sleep, and appetite, leading to yet more fatigue. And, of course, when the immune system is functioning less than optimally, there's a greater likelihood of additional infections. Dental infections are believed to be one kind of infection that can become chronic and give rise to this vicious cycle.

Mycoplasma and Other Organisms

One type of infection that seems to be common in people with FM and CFS is *mycoplasma*, very small bacteria (Nasralla, Haier, and Nicolson 1999). Mycoplasma differ from all other bacteria in that they have no cell wall, enabling them to invade cells, tissues, and blood—resulting in systemic infections in numerous organs. They do this by infecting white blood cells and using them for transportation throughout the body. Mycoplasma are able to lie dormant for a long time and "hide" from the immune system. This can lead to the activation of the immune system without achievement of the desired results. It's believed (Baseman and Tully 1997) that when mycoplasma attach to a cell and cause it to rupture, they hold onto a piece of the cell wall and may thus trigger the immune system to attack the cell, resulting in autoimmune dysfunction.

Suboptimal functioning of the immune system can also lead to overgrowth of fungi, bacteria, and parasites that are normally present in the digestive tracts of our bodies (Galland 1998). When these organisms, such as candida and giardia, proliferate, they tend to activate allergic responses, which in turn lead to many of the symptoms seen in FM and CFS.

Suhadolnik et al. (1997) found a specific defective immune system pathway in people with CFS that creates a vulnerability to opportunistic infections such as Epstein-Barr (EBV), human herpes virus-6 (HHV-6), enteroviruses, Coxsackie, and cytomegalovirus (CMV), as well as to overgrowth of bacteria such as mycoplasma and chlamydia. It appears that there may be a problem with an enzyme called *human leukocyte elastase* (HLE), which breaks down two proteins, *RNase-L* and

Stat-1 (Knox et al. 2004), required for white cells to properly respond to invading organisms. People with CFS display greatly increased levels of RNase-L, and it has been observed that the form of RNase-L seen in people with CFS is a smaller one than the norm. Stat-1 levels have been found to be low in some people with CFS and high in others (Knox et al. 2004). Recent research has also identified parainfluenza virus-5 as a potential cause of CFS; it has been found in a high percentage of people tested and is known to attack the Stat-1 protein (National CFIDS Foundation 2006).

Immune Response Inhibitors

Caffeine, alcohol, and refined sugar can all suppress immune response, as can environmental toxins, some medications, and poor diet. Chronic stress and strong emotions, even those that are suppressed, can also impact the effectiveness of the immune system. The brain and the different components of the immune system communicate with each other through the use of chemicals and nerve impulses to mount a well-coordinated defense. This interface makes it possible for thoughts and emotions to impact the immune system. For example, in several studies natural killer cells were found to be less active in people under stress, and helper T cells were reduced as well (Connor and Leonard 1998). Similarly, more antibodies to herpes viruses (some of which are implicated in FM and CFS) have been found in people under stress—considered an indicator that cell-based forms of immunity weren't operating properly and the body had to resort to more general immune responses.

This pattern also appears to correlate with unhappiness and other negative emotions (discussed in Collinge 1993). People who reported feeling more joy were able to mount better cellular defenses than those who were neutral or unhappy. This was found to be true even when these emotions came from simply watching movies. Levels of *endorphins*— natural painkillers that are activated by positive emotions and assist in the regulation of the immune system—were found to be low in patients with FM and CFS (Panerai et al. 2002). In one study, people who were able to find meaning in the loss of a loved one displayed increased immune response in the form of natural killer cells when compared to those who could not (Bower et al. 2003).

Immune response can be measured by standard lab tests of T cells, antibodies, and other immune system components.

Repair of Free Radical Damage

Our bodies are made up of molecules and molecules are made up of atoms. You may recall that every atom has a nucleus around which electrons orbit. Every orbit has a specific number of spaces for electrons. An electrically neutral atom is one that has the full complement of electrons in its outer orbit. If an atom's outer orbit isn't full, the atom is electrically charged and will correct this either by taking an electron from another atom, giving one up, or sharing one with another atom, thus creating a bond between the two. Charged atoms are known as *ions*. Minerals are transported in the blood as ions. Molecules, too, can be charged; a few of these, known as *free radicals*, have the power to damage other vital molecules, such as DNA.

The Causes and Consequences of Free Radical Damage

An excess of free radicals can result from a lack of nutrients needed to maintain balance as well as from environmental pollutants, pesticides, radiation, cigarette smoking, consumption of trans fats, and to some degree, from the natural aging process itself. An excess of free radicals can also be initiated by increases in metabolism rates—such as occurs in athletic training, while healing from an illness, or from eating excessive calories.

With too many free radicals, cell damage—called *oxidative stress* or *free radical damage*—can result. Depending on what cells are affected, health consequences can be substantial. There are strong indicators that oxidative stress is a major factor in FM and CFS. For example, levels of *malondialdehyde* (MDA)—a marker of free radical damage—have been found to be significantly higher in people with FM and CFS than in people without these syndromes, and *superoxide dismutase* (SOD)—a marker of antioxidant capacity—significantly lower (Bagis et al. 2005). It's believed this may indicate that FM and CFS are disorders of the balance of oxidation and antioxidants in the body. Fulle et al. (2000) found that oxidative damage to muscle tissue might be one cause of postexertional fatigue in people with FM and CFS, while Jammes et al. (2005) found increased use of the body's antioxidants during and after exercise in people with FM and CFS compared to healthy people. Kennedy et al. (2005) also found a correlation between raised levels of oxidative stress and the postexertional malaise and joint pain found in FM and CFS.

Antioxidants

The nutrients that control the chain reaction of free radical damage are called *antioxidants*. The best known antioxidants are vitamins C and E. Antioxidants offer up their own electrons so that free radicals no longer need to steal from other molecules. As you can imagine, antioxidants are very useful to have around. This is one of the reasons it's so important to eat fruits and vegetables—they are our primary source of antioxidants.

Glutathione, a protein that serves an antioxidant function in the cells, plays an important role in both detoxification and mitochondrial maintenance. People with FM and CFS often have low levels of glutathione. Van Konynenburg (2004) believes that depletion of glutathione is a central cause of FM and CFS.

Some specialized labs offer antioxidant testing profiles.

Circulation

The major function of your circulatory system is transportation. *Arteries* are vessels that carry blood away from the heart; *veins* are vessels that return blood to the heart. The heart is the pump that drives this system. We've already discussed how blood carries oxygen to tissues to be used and carbon dioxide to the lungs to be expelled. In addition, blood carries nutrients from the digestive tract to the cells in your body. Blood is also responsible for carrying waste products from the normal processes of your body to the kidneys, to be excreted in urine. Blood is also the principal carrier for hormones and an important conduit of the immune system.

Circulatory Dysfunction

A number of factors influence the functioning of your circulatory system. Because this system is basically a pump with some rather sophisticated pipes, major problems can result from a breakdown of the pump (when the heart doesn't work as it should), or a blockage in the pipes. However, these problems are rare in FM and CFS.

Rate of Circulation

The rate at which your heart pumps blood is determined by a number of factors, including your activity level, emotions, and environmental temperature. These functions are controlled by your *hypothalamus*, a part of the brain that regulates the brain chemicals that cause blood vessels in your muscles and skin to constrict or dilate. Hypothalamus function is frequently compromised in people with FM and CFS.

People with FM and CFS often have cold extremities and report feeling cold when others around them do not. Research has found capillary abnormalities and decreased blood flow in the extremities of people with FM or CFS (Morf et al. 2005). Elvin and colleagues (2006) also found decreased blood flow to muscles of people with FM and CFS during exercise. They hypothesize that this might be a cause of the pain experienced during exercise.

Blood Pressure

Another circulatory problem can be blood pressure that's either too low or too high. Blood pressure is influenced by how much blood you have as well as the thickness of your blood—thicker blood offers more resistance in small arteries and can eventually cause blockages in capillaries. As we saw in the section on respiration, a dysregulation of the coagulation process in the blood, causing it to be thicker than normal, is often found in people with FM and CFS. This can lead to excess deposits of *fibrin*—sometimes called "nature's bandage"—on the walls of the blood vessels, making it harder for blood to pass through (Berg et al. 1999). Ironically, even though this coagulation process is triggered by the body in order to help fight infections, the same process can make it harder to fight infections, because viruses and bacteria can "hide" under the fibrin (Kaplan 2001).

High blood pressure isn't common in people with FM and CFS. However, people with FM and CFS often have low blood pressure—or sometimes blood pressure that's unusually variable (Naschitz et al. 2005). Blood pressure that's too low is problematic: without sufficient force, the body can't get blood to your brain effectively. When the brain is deprived of blood, there are significant problems in both the short term—such as a tendency to faint—and in the long term—such as fatigue, weakness, and a lowered ability to think and carry out other higher order brain functions.

Dehydration can increase a tendency toward low blood pressure. If you already have low blood pressure, it may be temporarily worsened by eating because digestion requires your body to send blood to your core, leaving your periphery with less blood flow. This can be even worse with sugary foods because they can induce functional *hypoglycemia*—low blood sugar, common in people with FM and CFS—which can lead to problems with your brain's use of glucose, its main energy source, thus further impairing your brain's functioning.

Blood Composition

The proportion of red blood cells in your blood is important, because red blood cells contain hemoglobin, the substance that carries oxygen. Low hemoglobin is a form of anemia, and very common in FM and CFS. As we have seen, a lack of hemoglobin will cause cells to be partially deprived of oxygen, and as a result, you may become weak and tired. When blood cells are lost through menstrual or other forms of bleeding, some of the iron in your system is lost, making it hard for your body to produce hemoglobin. Other causes of low hemoglobin include an inability of bone marrow to incorporate iron—sometimes seen with chronic infection—and a lack of certain nutrients, most notably vitamin B_{12} and folate. Blood tests are used to assess both the level of hemoglobin and some of its common causes.

Mitral Valve Prolapse

Another circulatory problem that people with FM and CFS are prone to is *mitral valve prolapse* (MVP), an abnormality in one of the valves of the heart. Although the valve is supposed to allow blood to flow in only one direction, with MVP the valve allows some blood to flow back into the heart. This can cause palpitations, and in some cases lead to infection (Pellegrino et al. 1989).

Cardiac Insufficiency

Paul Cheney has suggested that CFS symptoms result from the body's prioritizing blood flow to essential organs and tissues in an attempt to compensate for reduced blood output due to a damaged heart muscle (Sieverling 2005). Heart tissue may be damaged by viral infection or an accumulation of mercury (Frustaci et al. 1999) among other things. Cheney believes that cardiac output is a highly reliable predictor of degree of disability in people with CFS.

While the Cheney theory is compelling, it hasn't been published yet in a peer-reviewed medical journal, so there has been no opportunity as of yet for other researchers to respond to the accuracy of the model.

Diagnosing Heart Problems

Problems with the circulatory system can be diagnosed in a number of ways: checking your pulse for abnormally fast or slow heartbeats, listening to the heart for characteristic sounds that indicate MVP or a blockage, stress tests on a treadmill, ultrasounds, CT scans, echocardiograms and other imaging techniques, blood tests for hemoglobin, and measuring blood pressure when standing and sitting and in the arm and the leg, as well as by symptoms such as chest pain or certain kinds of leg pain.

Detoxification

Our bodies are routinely exposed to a large number of toxic substances, in the food we eat, the air we breathe, the water we drink and bathe in, and the products we use. We encounter hundreds of chemicals in our everyday lives that are possible toxins. In addition, our bodies produce toxins in the course of their normal functioning. We have a number of systems in place to protect us from the effects of all of these toxins.

We have seen how the waste products of individual cells are eliminated through the blood, the lymphatic system, and the lungs. We have also discussed how the bowel serves to eliminate waste from our food. The liver is also a major player in the detoxification process, not only serving as a filter for all of the blood in your body, but also turning toxic substances into less toxic ones that can be safely eliminated. Your kidneys are also responsible for filtering toxic substances from your body. In this process they also carefully regulate the amount of water and certain other substances—such as calcium, magnesium, sodium, phosphorus, and potassium—in your body. When the kidneys and liver don't quite eliminate all of the toxins, your skin can serve as an additional organ of elimination. In women, menstruation serves as another channel for the elimination of toxins.

Toxicity in FM and CFS

Goldberg (1998) and many other FM and CFS experts suggest that excess toxicity may be the main cause of FM and CFS. Excess toxicity may be caused by excessive exposure to toxins, a reduced ability to detoxify, or both. It may be exacerbated by an inflammation of the intestines that allows food to pass into the bloodstream before it is fully digested, causing food to be treated by the body as a toxin. The symptoms of toxic buildup can be nearly anything, and encompass the main symptoms of FM and CFS: brain fog, low energy, pain, headaches, skin rash, etc.

Mercury and aluminum toxicities have been found in people with FM and CFS (Shanklin et al. 2000), as has aspartame toxicity (Smith et al. 2001). Van Konynenburg (2004) hypothesizes that depletion of glutathione—a depletion which is very common in people with FM or CFS—is a major cause of the excess mercury seen in people with FM or CFS.

Assessing Kidney and Liver Dysfunction

Liver dysfunction is usually assessed through the use of blood tests to measure certain enzymes that are normally confined to the liver but can leak into the blood when the liver is damaged. Standard blood tests can also measure levels of substances such as bilirubin, creatinine, and blood urea nitrogen—which are all byproducts of various metabolic processes, and can give an indication of liver and kidney function. Kidney function is usually measured through urine tests. Some less well-known tests are also available that challenge the body's detoxification process by means of some common substances that are ingested; the body's outputs in the saliva and urine are then measured.

Hormonal Balance

Just as neurotransmitters serve as chemical messengers that control many of the body's functions, hormones, too, work to regulate many of the functions of the body. The nervous system and the *endocrine* or hormonal system work together to keep each other balanced.

Hormones are produced by glands. Hormones may act locally, near where they are made, or they may travel to other parts of the body to exert their influence. The following is a very brief overview of the main parts of the endocrine system:

The *hypothalamus* region of the brain is involved in regulating the functions of the pituitary gland.

The *pituitary gland*—often thought of as the master gland because it regulates the functioning of the other glands—is located at the base of the brain; it secretes hormones that regulate the thyroid and adrenal glands as well as the growth and development of bone, muscle, and the sex organs.

The *adrenal glands*, located above the kidneys, secrete hormones that are involved in the fight-or-flight response of the sympathetic nervous system.

The *parathyroid glands*, located above the adrenal glands, are involved in calcium regulation.

The *pancreas* manages the concentration of glucose in the blood.

The *pineal gland* regulates sleep-wake cycles.

The Hypothalamic-Pituitary-Adrenal Axis

The *hypothalamic-pituitary-adrenal axis* (HPA axis) is the body's stress management system, for both physical and emotional stress; some believe it's also the body's energy regulation mechanism. Most FM and CFS experts agree that HPA dysfunction is a central component of FM and CFS. When you experience stress, a series of actions is set off by the endocrine glands, beginning in the hypothalamus and leading to the secretion of the hormone *cortisol*. (Along the way, other hormones, involved in pain suppression, reproductive function, blood pressure and volume, and potassium-sodium balance in the blood, are also released.) Cortisol acts to increase the metabolism of glucose and suppress the immune system, the reproductive system, and digestion. Thus the HPA axis is involved—directly or indirectly—in bodily functions as diverse as motivation and mood, blood volume and pressure, fear response, memory, body temperature, appetite, growth and regeneration, sex drive and reproductive function, pain management, metabolism, and immunity.

Typically, cortisol production is maintained within certain upper and lower limits, allowing for both an apt response to current stress and a timely return to normal levels. Your level of cortisol normally follows a predictable pattern throughout the day; this is called a *circadian rhythm*. In people with FM and CFS, however, the HPA axis is underactive and the level of cortisol is generally lower and less variable, following a different daily pattern (McLean et al. 2005). There are also some indications of circadian abnormalities of another hormone, called *adrenocorticotropic hormone* (ACTH) (Di Giorgio et al. 2005).

Chronic Stress and Adrenal Function

During an acute stressor it's good to shut down nonessential systems to allow your body to act quickly to get you out of danger. However, if these nonessential systems are deferred for a long time, your body can start to break down. It's believed that this process of breakdown may explain many of the symptoms of FM and CFS.

A prolonged activation of the stress system can cause it to be overtaxed and unable to do its job. Almost half of a sample of people suffering from CFS showed mild signs of adrenal failure as well as atrophy of the adrenal glands (Scott, Teh, et al. 1999). If HPA axis changes continue for a long time, they may also alter the brain's ability to adapt to changing levels of stress, eventually leaving a person without an adequate stress response in times of need. In some ways, people with FM and CFS must thus deal with the effects of both too much cortisol and not enough cortisol. You will notice that this parallels the process we discussed in the section on the immune system, where the body's response is both underactive and overactive.

Chronic Stress and Growth Hormone

Growth hormone production is one of the nonessential systems that underfunction when stress is sustained for long periods of time. People with FM and CFS tend to have lower levels of growth hormone (Paiva et al. 2002). In adults, the effects of lower levels of growth hormone include poor general health, increased fat/decreased muscle, low energy, impaired cognition, depression, reduced skin thickness, reduced exercise capacity, reduced cardiac output, reduced plasma volume, and cold intolerance.

Emotions and Stress

Your perception of a situation affects how much of a stress response it can trigger. Most people who develop FM and CFS have experienced significantly stressful events, such as an illness, accident, or psychosocial stressors. Those who feel more hopeless and less in control of the stress appear to be the ones who develop the HPA axis insufficiency. The HPA axis appears to be activated first by an acute stressor, but is then maintained over the long term, possibly as a result of specific emotional attitudes (McBeth et al. 2005).

Chronic Stress and Thyroid Function

People with FM and CFS have been found to have lowered thyroid function—an important finding also suggestive of a blunted HPA axis response (Jefferies 1994). The effects of low thyroid function include fatigue, low energy, lowered metabolic rate, and cold extremities; many patients with low thyroid functioning also complain of shortness of breath (Lowe 2005).

Murphy et al. (2004) found differences in levels of the hormone progesterone in normal controls and people with CFS. Lee, Hanley, and Hopkins (1999) hypothesize that an imbalance of progesterone may be responsible for many of the symptoms of FM and CFS through its influence on other hormones that affect the thyroid gland, nerve transmission, calcium metabolism, mood, and other functions.

Assessing HPA Axis Dysfunction

HPA axis problems can be detected through standard and specialized lab tests of cortisol and other hormones. Unfortunately, problems with thyroid function can't easily be assessed through the use of standard blood tests—levels of thyroid hormones can test as being within or at the margins of the normal reference range, even when the impairment in thyroid function is significant. Some labs offer a comprehensive thyroid panel more likely to detect the kinds of thyroid problems that co-occur with FM and CFS. Sometimes these subtle differences can also be assessed through the use of a resting basal body temperature test (Sehnert and Croft 1996).

Structural Alignment and Balance

For many people with FM (and probably many with CFS as well, although this is less well documented), a trauma to the body preceded their illness and seemed to trigger it (Buskila et al. 1997). Because of this, increasing attention is being paid to the problems resulting from an accident or injury that has impacted the skeletal system, and how this might lead to a systemic illness such as FM or CFS.

There are five segments of the spine: the cervical spine at the top, then the thoracic and lumbar segments, followed by the bony sacrum and coccyx. The *spinal canal* is the channel enclosed by your vertebrae. The nerves of the central and peripheral nervous system pass through the spinal canal, bathed in cerebrospinal fluid. Because they fit quite snugly in this narrow canal, poor alignment of the bones of the spine can result in compressions and blockages that compromise nerve impulse transmission. This often happens on a very subtle level, and is common following an accident or injury. The type of dysfunction that results depends on which segment of the spine is affected. Pain may be localized at that place on the spine or felt further afield, in the places that the nerves connect to. It's believed that this process may be a central cause of symptoms in some people with FM and CFS, and that these people might comprise a distinct subgroup of FM and CFS (Heffez et al. 2004).

Osteoporosis—the loss of density in the bones—is also found in some people with FM and CFS (Swezey and Adams 1999). Although there's no evidence of a direct link between osteoporosis and FM or CFS, people with FM and CFS are known to display imbalances in calcium and magnesium metabolism; this could be the link. Another possible cause is the sustained lack of activity that results from the pain and fatigue of FM and CFS.

Chiari Malformation

Another very small subgroup of FM and CFS patients has been identified as suffering from *Chiari malformation*—when a part of the brain tissue extends down into the spinal cord, causing compression of the nerves and restriction of the flow of cerebrospinal fluid. Chiari malformations are seen more frequently among people diagnosed with FM and CFS than in the normal population, but the relationship between the syndromes is not clear at this time (Benzel et al. 2005).

Trigger Points

Another musculoskeletal phenomenon seen in people with FM or CFS is the presence of myofascial *trigger points*—small knots that develop in a muscle when it's injured or overworked. As a defense against injury, muscle and *fascia*—a weblike film of connective tissue that surrounds your muscles and organs—tighten up and limit the range of motion in that area. When one area of the body develops trigger points, the restriction in movement of that body part can then cause another body part to compensate, causing more trigger points to form. It's not unusual to have trigger points in many parts of the body. When a trigger point is stimulated, pain is "referred" along predictable pathways mapped out by Simons et al. (1998) in their classic medical textbook on trigger points. It is believed that trigger points are involved in most cases of chronic pain.

Many people with FM and CFS have active trigger points. One of the more common sites of trigger points in people with FM and CFS is the muscles surrounding the temporomandibular joint (TMJ) of the jaw. In fact, one study found that 87 percent of patients with FM had problems with this joint (Manfredini et al. 2004).

Posture and Balance

According to an article in *Fibromyalgia Network* (1995), there may be a relationship between some of the symptoms of FM and posture.

Herbert Gordon says that when we carry our weight incorrectly we cause damage to our muscles and ligaments—which can then set off a cascade of problems, including greatly decreased efficiency of our energy, and a resulting increase in pain. One study documented different patterns of muscle usage in women with FM (Pierrynowski, Tiidus, and Galea 2005). Physical therapist Mary Biancalana has observed that people with FM tend to use secondary muscles to accomplish work their major muscles should be doing, which can be exhausting.

Assessing Musculoskeletal Problems

Some of the problems described in this section can be diagnosed by a chiropractor trained in the evaluation of spinal alignment and body mechanics. Some movement specialists—such as teachers of the Alexander technique or structural integration—can evaluate patterns of posture and inefficient movement. Problems with the spine can be evaluated by magnetic resonance imaging (MRI), CT scans, myelograms, and measures of the flow of cerebrospinal fluid. Osteoporosis can be assessed with a special kind of X-ray test used for measuring bone density.

Sleep and Restoration

High quality sleep is necessary for vibrant health. During sleep the body repairs itself. Sleep also promotes growth and development and the consolidation of learning. The onset, duration, and quality of sleep are determined by environmental factors—such as the light and dark portions of the day—emotions, hormones, and other internal physiological factors. Pain, medications, alcohol, and even some foods can affect sleep.

Optimal sleep consists of defined periods of time spent in five different stages. Each of the stages appears to serve a distinct function. If you don't get the proper proportions of each stage, a multitude of symptoms can result, including, among others, fatigue, excessive daytime sleepiness, irritability, anxiety, depression, pain, memory problems, poor coordination, problems with concentration and attention, and possibly blood sugar handling problems.

Sleep Disorders

In addition to *insomnia*—a difficulty falling asleep and/or staying asleep—there are a number of other sleep disorders common among people with FM and CFS. These include disorders of movement during sleep, disorders of the stages of sleep, and disorders of the process of breathing during sleep.

Disorders of Movement During Sleep

Periodic leg movements of sleep (PLMS) is the nighttime variant of restless leg syndrome—a nearly unbearable impulse to move the legs due to unusual sensations described as tingly or crawly. During sleep, involuntary leg movements result in waking the person up or disrupting the deepest levels of sleep. The cause of PLMS is unknown, but the condition appears to be associated with poor circulation, anemia, kidney disorders, alcoholism, vitamin and mineral deficiencies (MacFarlane et al. 1996), and an inability of part of the brain to properly utilize iron (Connor et al. 2003). It seems that problems with the neurotransmitter dopamine are central to this disorder—it's relieved by medications that increase the availability of dopamine (Allen et al. 2004). Some people have reported PLMS as a side effect of certain antidepressant medications.

Disorders of the Stages of Sleep

The sleep stage problem most common among people with FM and CFS is *alpha-delta sleep*—when more superficial levels of sleep intrude on deeper levels, thus limiting the time spent in deep sleep. People with FM and CFS also have fewer *sleep spindles*—characteristic patterns of brain waves associated with normal sleep (Landis et al. 2004).

Disorders of the Process of Breathing During Sleep

Disorders of the process of breathing during sleep are referred to as *sleep apnea*. People with sleep apnea stop breathing for very brief periods of time while asleep, causing them to awaken as many as hundreds of times in a night. This can be caused by the physical obstruction of the airway, a problem with the brain's signaling, or both. People with FM or CFS have higher than average rates of sleep apnea (Gold et al. 2004). Alvarez and colleagues (1996) believe that sleep apnea may account for some of the musculoskeletal pain experienced with FM and CFS.

It seems clear that the disordered sleep seen in FM and CFS isn't directly caused by emotional factors or pain. Although these elements can exacerbate sleep problems, sleep difficulties in FM and CFS appear to be related to the same kinds of biochemical problems that cause the syndromes' other symptoms, according to Yunus and Aldag (1996); the syndromes' emotional difficulties appear to arise from the sleep deprivation (Lentz et al. 1999).

Because of sleep disorders, people with FM and CFS have difficulty getting enough *delta*—or deep—sleep. In one study, people who didn't have FM or CFS but were purposely deprived of delta sleep for a few nights developed many of the symptoms of FM and CFS, indicating that lack of delta sleep may be a cause of symptoms in people who do have FM or CFS (Lentz et al. 1999).

During delta sleep the amount of growth hormone released by the pituitary gland is increased, to facilitate repair and regeneration of muscles (Moldofsky et al. 1975). Growth hormone triggers the body to make growth factors such as somatomedin C (also called insulin-like growth factor 1). Some studies show that FM sufferers display abnormally low levels of this substance, while people with CFS display higher levels than normal (Bennett et al. 1997). However, other research doesn't confirm this trend (Buchwald, Umali, and Stene 1996). Bennett et al. (1997) believe that low levels of somatomedin C may be a cause of the muscle pain and fatigue commonly seen in fibromyalgia.

It's also during delta sleep that the immune system becomes more active, so without proper sleep immunity can be lowered.

Assessing Sleep Disorders

You can be fairly certain that all is not well with your sleep if, even after sleeping eight hours, you wake up tired. This is extremely common in FM and CFS. Sleep disorders can be assessed by *polysomnography*—a process of monitoring a variety of bodily processes, such as pulse, respiration, muscle tension, and electric activity in the brain, while you sleep in a laboratory setting. This is referred to as a *sleep study*.

Emotional Response

Emotional health has two parts: baseline emotional functioning—the way you feel when everything is okay; and coping methods—the way you feel when life brings you challenges.

Healthy Emotional Response

Good baseline functioning involves a balance of goal-oriented and relaxing activities. Some people are too focused on work goals, child rearing, perfecting a sport, etc. Other people are unable to activate themselves enough to achieve even basic goals like taking care of themselves and their home. No matter how relaxing your downtime or how successfully you achieve goals, an overfocus on one or the other isn't as healthy as balance. People with FM or CFS tend to be overly goal-oriented.

Another aspect of healthy baseline functioning is the ability to experience a full range of emotions, both "good" ones and "bad" ones. In other words, it's a normal part of good emotional health to feel angry, jealous, afraid, and confused sometimes. Feeling happy or elated all the time isn't realistic; life involves loss, disappointment, conflict, and other unhappy things. It doesn't make sense to face these events with happiness. However, if you both face these events with genuine emotion and really feel your more pleasant emotions, you may very well experience your life as happy over the long run.

In people with FM and CFS there's a slight tendency to be out of touch with parts of the range of emotion, or unaware of or split off from emotions in general. One problem that has been observed with people with FM is that they don't easily maintain positive emotions in the face of stressors. This suggests that these people lack the emotional resources to bounce back when things go wrong (Zautra et al. 2005). Zautra and colleagues also found that people with FM tend to withdraw from social interactions when stressed more than some other people with pain do, and that while stress didn't increase levels of pain, it did increase levels of fatigue.

Good emotional health also involves being able to be in relationships that are mutually satisfying. To accomplish this, you must be able to both say what you need and listen empathically when others tell you about their feelings. When a relationship centers too much on one person, it's not healthy. A truly reciprocal relationship usually requires reasonably good self-esteem. Some people with FM and CFS have low self-esteem; however, it's not clear whether this is a cause or an effect.

Emotions in the Face of Adversity

When really bad things happen—particularly those over which we feel we have no control—our emotional wellness is challenged. We all have different ways of coping with adversity; some ways are more practical than others. Some people cope by taking action to change the situation. Some people cope by expressing their feelings or seeking help from others. Some people cope by avoiding the situation. As you can guess, avoidant coping isn't ideal, although it does come in handy sometimes. Most people use a combination of emotion-focused and action-focused coping.

One kind of avoidant coping involves converting emotions into physical symptoms. This isn't done consciously. In fact, many of these people—often referred to as *somatizers*—initially don't believe they're doing it. It's said that people with FM and CFS tend to be somatizers. However, to be diagnosed as a somatizer, a person must have a number of "medically unexplained" symptoms. Because symptoms of FM and CFS have been considered medically unexplained—even though this isn't entirely accurate—people with FM and CFS have often been incorrectly classified as somatizers (e.g., Allen et al. 2002), making these findings regarding somatizers difficult to interpret.

Similarly, the very concept of somatization begs the question of how connected the mind and body really are. If, as seems to be the case, emotions directly affect the nervous system and the endocrine system, it doesn't make sense to say that illnesses caused or exacerbated by stress are any less "medical." We may all be somatizers to varying degrees. For the most part, medical professionals have not yet considered the implications of this.

Childhood Experiences and FM and CFS

Certain elements of childhood history are shared by many people with FM and CFS. These include rape (Ciccone et al. 2005) and childhood sexual abuse (Walker et al. 1997). Not only are people with FM and CFS more likely to have a history of abuse than the general population, but people with this history are also more likely to experience more severe pain, both from FM as well as from other causes (Alexander et al. 1998). There are some indicators that the increased pain level seen in abuse survivors is due, at least in part, to the effects of the depression that follows the abuse (De Civita, Bernatsky, and Dobkin 2004).

While depression is a significant part of the experience of FM and CFS, brain imaging studies suggest depression itself doesn't directly affect the level of pain a person experiences (Giesecke et al. 2005). Rather, people with FM or CFS who are more depressed tend to experience more unpleasantness associated with the pain, as indicated by the activation of parts of the brain involved in processing unpleasantness but not pain. This isn't typical at all for other people with pain (Giesecke et al. 2005).

It has been hypothesized that post-traumatic stress disorder may be the connection between abuse experiences and the onset of FM and CFS (Ciccone et al. 2005). Post-traumatic stress disorder, among other things, keeps the body in a constant state of stress, which can then trigger the neuroendocrine changes discussed earlier. In support of this, people with histories of abuse have been found to have altered cortisol responses (Weissbecker et al. 2006). Important, groundbreaking work on the lasting biochemical effects of abuse has been done by Allan Schore (1999).

Depression: Cause or Effect?

You may have heard somebody say that FM and CFS are physical manifestations of depression, and that if you rid yourself of your depression, you'll regain your health. Actually, there are strong indications that the relationship between depression and illness is just the opposite: that depression comes as a reaction to the illness and the limitations it places on what you can do. When you have to drastically change activities that form a large part of how you define yourself, depression can result. Changes in what you can do can also change the nature of your relationships with loved ones—which can give rise to a mixture of emotions, including depression and anxiety.

A study conducted by the Centers for Disease Control (Axe et al. 2004) found no differences between the rates of depression in people with CFS and healthy people. However, just as in healthy people, some people with FM and CFS have had depression and panic attacks prior to the onset of their physical symptoms. Hudson and colleagues (1992) hypothesize that sometimes the same physical problems can give rise to both the depression or panic attacks and the FM or CFS. It's possible that there's a common underlying cause for both found in a genetic predisposition to problems with the serotonin system (Raphael et al. 2004).

It's important to know as well that some of the elements out of balance in your body will also directly lead to symptoms such as depression. A good example is an underactive thyroid—doctors have known for years that depression is a symptom of hypothyroidism. Similarly, if you have hypoglycemia, you might feel panicky; if you have a problem with energy production, you might feel depressed; and so on. Adrenal fatigue can also lead to both depression and anxiety, and sleep problems are a well-known source of depressed mood.

Assessing Emotional Wellness

Just as there are many ways of defining emotional wellness, there are many ways of measuring it. For our purposes here you can ask yourself whether you had satisfying relationships and adequate pleasure in your life before you started feeling ill, and whether you were able to cope well with adversity. Another way of looking at this is to consider whether you were relatively free of depression, anxiety, obsessive thinking, and feeling driven. For some people this may be experienced more as not feeling fully in touch with themselves. If you're unsure of whether your emotional functioning is problematic, a psychologist can usually do a thorough assessment in a few sessions.

Spiritual Wellness

By spiritual wellness I mean a general sense of purpose and meaning in your life and a connection to some source of replenishment for your soul. For some people, this entails having a way to understand things like what happens after we die, why bad things happen to good people, how to define right and wrong, and the best way to live.

These things can be achieved in many different ways, and may entail religious practices such as prayer, meditation, or participation in rituals. You may also find your sense of meaning and source of replenishment in other ways, such as being near the ocean, being around children, or having quiet time for yourself. If all is not well in this area, you may experience depression, alienation, and feelings of being tapped out, overwhelmed, and hopeless.

Balance of Subtle Energies

Throughout history many different cultures have had ways of understanding what has been called universal life force, life energy, chi, ki, reiki, or prana. A general definition of this life energy is that it's the subtle essence that enlivens us and provides every kind of energy, the difference between a live person and a deceased one. There are many ways of thinking about how this life energy works, but the general idea is that it flows along certain pathways in the body. If all is well, its flow is smooth and unimpeded. Sometimes, however, this life energy becomes blocked or compacted and loses its vitality.

When life energy isn't flowing freely, a person may feel tired or lack energy. Emotional problems can also result. There may also be a sense of a lack of integration of mind, body, and spirit. In people with FM and CFS, it is said that the life energy has become weakened, and that this is the source of the fatigue and other symptoms. The weakening of life energy can be caused by physical, emotional, or spiritual factors. Some people seem to have a gift for sensing subtle energies and can assess their levels and flow.

CHAPTER 3

Orchestrating Your Health Care

Choosing the right treatment for FM and CFS can be a challenge—
there are dozens of treatments available and deciding among them is like
comparing apples and oranges. In fact, it's often more like comparing
McIntosh apples and Fujis to grapefruit, tangelos, lemons, and bananas!
Here are some of the factors that make comparisons difficult:

■ Some approaches are more conventional; some are more
alternative.

■ Some are comprehensive and can address a wide range
of symptoms; some are targeted to just one or two
symptoms.

■ Some approaches require very little of you; some require
a lot—this can vary from simply swallowing a pill to a
complete lifestyle change.

■ Some approaches are based on an underlying philosophy that guides the entire treatment; some are purely
pragmatic, based on what works.

■ Some approaches are practiced by licensed professionals;
some approaches have no regulatory oversight.

■ How well an approach can be practiced at home without
the guidance of a health professional varies.

■ If a health professional's advice is needed, other factors
that vary include how frequently visits may be needed,

how much they cost, and whether they're covered by medical insurance.

- Some approaches have been studied for effectiveness; some have not.

- Some approaches are legitimate curative attempts; some are simply founded in a desire for profit or fame.

- Some approaches can be combined effectively; some conflict with each other.

So, how do you make your way through this maze of health care? Follow these four steps:

1. Learn about what kinds of dysfunction you are trying to correct. Chapter 2 has covered the information you need to make this determination.

2. Find out what approaches are available to treat the specific kinds of dysfunction you're experiencing. The rest of this book will cover most of the reasonable options for treating FM and CFS; each chapter will tell you which of the elements of health the approach focused on can be used to treat.

3. Decide which approach best suits your symptoms, your resources, and your preferences. The worksheet at the end of this chapter will help you pull together information from the different chapters.

4. Finally, for approaches that involve a practitioner of some kind, you must find one whom you trust. I offer some guidelines on making that decision in this chapter and will address specific aspects of it in the chapters on each of the different healing approaches.

Step 3 can be pretty tricky. Many people get stuck when it comes to deciding how many approaches to choose. Some people choose approaches that are redundant and waste time and money. Some choose approaches that can't address the full range of their symptoms. This often leaves people with a less than satisfactory result. However, with a clear system for information organization and decision making, you can get past the confusion and create your own plan for relief.

A System for Decision Making

Imagine a symphony orchestra. There are many different instruments. They all make music, but they make it in different ways: by moving a bow across strings, by blowing air into a tube, by banging on a tightly stretched skin, by causing a reed to vibrate. In order to make a beautiful piece of music, a conductor calls upon musicians to play their instruments in various combinations. Sometimes—very rarely—the whole orchestra plays in unison. Sometimes each section plays something different, making a sound all together that is very pleasant to hear. Sometimes a soloist is the only one playing. Sometimes a musician plays more than one instrument at different times during the piece, like a percussionist who plays the snare drum, cymbals, bass drum, tambourine, and triangle. Or two dozen violins might all play the same part—or the first and second violins harmonize. Flutes and oboes might team up to play the same melody. Some instruments, such as the trumpet, are good at being solo carriers of the tune, while others, such as the triangle, don't stand alone very well. A good conductor knows how to make the best use of the talents of each of the musicians in the orchestra.

Orchestrating your own health care is similar in many ways. Using one of the more comprehensive health care modalities that addresses all of your functions is like having the soloist carrying the piece of music. Choosing two approaches for one kind of dysfunction is like directing the oboe and the flute to play the same melody, with each adding their unique timbre. Addressing each symptom with a different approach is like allowing each section of the orchestra to contribute something different to the sound. Using a comprehensive approach, but adding in another approach to enhance it is like having a piano join a soloist's ongoing performance. Health professionals who use many different healing approaches are like the percussionist who seamlessly moves from one instrument to another.

All of these ways of making music are available to you. Your job is to orchestrate your own efforts and those of your providers so that the various functions disrupted in your body are addressed in a coherent way by one or more healing approaches. Because most people with FM and CFS have a broad range of dysfunction, this can typically be achieved in a number of ways—giving you the flexibility to choose from both alternative and mainstream approaches. You can also, within limits, have as much or as little assistance in your own care as you choose.

The following two stories show how this might work out in practice:

■ *Janet's Story*

Janet had fibromyalgia. Pain was a primary symptom for her—she ached all over and frequently got severe headaches. She also experienced fatigue, dizziness, weakness, and alternating constipation and diarrhea. She went to her physician for a checkup and blood work and made careful observations of her body and its patterns on her own. As a result she discovered that she didn't feel well after eating certain foods (digestive dysfunction), had a relative deficiency of magnesium and vitamin D (nutritional dysfunction), was low on hemoglobin (respiratory dysfunction), and lacked a sense of purpose and direction in her life (spiritual dysfunction).

After doing careful research on proper forms and doses, Janet decided to supplement her diet with magnesium, iron, and vitamin D to address her nutritional and respiratory dysfunctions. She also stopped eating foods she knew made her feel ill in order to give her digestive tract a chance to heal. After two months on this regimen, her weakness, fatigue, and dizziness were gone, and she had achieved partial relief of her pain. The headaches remained, as did most of her digestive problems. At this point, she decided to go on a food elimination diet to determine whether there were any other foods she was sensitive to. After educating herself about how to do this, she identified a number of other foods that were problematic and eliminated these from her diet as well. She started using licorice root and chamomile to help her digestive tract heal further. She also began taking a meditation class to manage stress and address her spiritual dysfunction. Four months later she felt well and was continuing to explore her spirituality.

■ Shirley's Story

Shirley had very severe fatigue and low energy; as a result she could no longer work. She often felt nauseated, and couldn't tolerate cold. She persistently had a slightly elevated temperature and a sore throat. She had a history of depression and had been taking an antidepressant for a year, so when she began to feel tired she chalked it up to a return of the depression. However, when the problems persisted, she realized that the persistent sore throat and fever meant she must also be experiencing immune system dysfunction. When her doctor sent her for a sleep study she learned that she also had sleep dysfunction in the form of periodic leg movements of sleep (PLMS).

Shirley had read that the medication she was taking could sometimes cause PLMS, so she worked with her doctor to reduce the medication. As a result, she was less tired but her depression became more severe and her moods more variable. She decided to visit a traditional Chinese medicine specialist. This specialist worked with her on balancing the energies in her body through the use of herbs, acupuncture, and moxibustion. She achieved relief of all of her symptoms and learned how to eat foods appropriate for her constitution and the season of the year. A few months later, when a relationship breakup triggered a return of her depression, she sought psychotherapy to learn drug-free approaches to maintaining her emotional wellness.

An approach like Janet's may make more sense for you if you live in a place where there aren't many holistic health practitioners or you prefer a self-care approach and have the ability to do some research into your treatment options. A path like Shirley's may be more appealing for you if you prefer to keep things simple by having one person coordinate most of your care, you're too ill or too brain-fogged to learn to carry out a self-care regimen, or human contact with a health care practitioner feels healing to you. In both cases, the women worked with the resources within themselves and their communities to craft a unique treatment plan for their patterns of dysfunction. Janet's approach was more like an orchestra with each instrument section contributing a different part of the whole piece of music, while Shirley's was more like a solo instrument lightly accented by other instruments. In both cases, the approaches resulted in beautiful music—symptom relief and restoration of proper function.

Combining Treatments

The chapters on the different healing modalities will provide you with the information you need to decide if it's a good idea to combine different approaches. For example, because both certain herbs and massage therapy can be used to manage stress, these two approaches may appropriately be combined if more than one approach to relaxation is needed; then again, massage alone may be able to do the job. Some approaches are dangerous to combine. For example, if you're taking certain antidepressants and you add in *Saint-John's-wort*—an herb that has a similar biochemical effect in the body—the combination can be dangerously potent. Some combinations may also simply lead to redundancy, such as a combination of traditional Chinese medicine and ayurveda, two healing approaches that treat many of the same symptoms from slightly different perspectives.

The goal is to orchestrate your own treatment, either by selecting one approach that addresses all or most of your symptoms, or by combining several complementary approaches to address all of your needs. Choosing from many health care approaches gives you the flexibility to work with those you have access to or those you prefer. And taking charge of your own health care will give you a sense of control over your situation—which is healing in itself, as it addresses the emotional response function. The more of your dysfunctions you address, the more likely you are to recover. Your body has a better chance of self-healing once the burden of dysfunction is reduced.

How Do You Know if It Will Work?

Nobody can say for sure whether you'll find success with any given treatment. However, you can improve your ability to make good predictions by considering both anecdotal evidence and scientific research.

Anecdotal Evidence

Anecdotal evidence basically amounts to others' personal experiences with different approaches. There are obvious problems to basing treatment decisions on anecdotal evidence: not only must we depend on the reliability of the person providing the information, they must be appropriately similar to ourselves. The accuracy of the anecdotal evidence can be

influenced both by a tendency to wishful thinking in the person report-
ing the information, and by a tendency in us to exaggerate the positive
aspects of what we're hearing due to a strong desire to find a solution.

Scientific Research

Research reports aren't always completely reliable either. For example,
a bias toward certain results can be introduced when studies are funded
or conducted by people who stand to profit from those results. Also,
although an approach may have been found effective for some symptoms,
it may not be effective for the specific problem you're experiencing. For
example, although antidepressant medications are pretty effective for
managing pain caused by neurotransmitter imbalances, if your pain is
caused by poor posture, antidepressants may not be effective for you.
Also, research studies may disagree, one study showing an approach
effective while another study finds the same approach ineffective. And
research studies may be unclear: it may look like a treatment has caused
improvement when that improvement is actually due to another cause.
Additionally, some treatments don't get researched because nobody has
the time or the money to carry the research out—research is expensive and sometimes funding sources prefer to stick with less innovative
approaches until anecdotal evidence accumulates.

Sometimes scientific research is also skewed by a mismatch between
how an approach works and traditional methods of research. For example,
standard research methods sometimes require that a health professional
be unaware of which treatment is being applied to his or her patient—or
that the same treatment is applied to every patient. But this is contrary to
the very essence of some approaches, e.g., massage and acupuncture. And
even if a large, reputable body of research demonstrates the effectiveness
of a given approach for research participants, it may not be effective for
every patient. This is particularly true for complex syndromes like FM
and CFS. Designing an individualized treatment regimen requires art
as well as science.

Finding What's Right For You

So, how do you find an approach that you can trust to work? One
way is to select an approach that has a long history of effectiveness in

many kinds of situations, with many kinds of people. This will overcome some—but not all—of the problems that come from relying on smaller amounts of anecdotal evidence. For example, it may be easier to trust that you'll find safe relief with traditional Chinese medicine—which has been around for centuries—than with an approach that is brand new. Another way is to wait until multiple research studies with impeccable methods all point in the same direction. This will eliminate most of the problems of relying on anecdotal evidence—but requires that you wait until an approach has been around for quite a while before being able to benefit from it. Another way is to use your own intuition about an approach, based on either the appeal of the underlying concept or your sense of the reliability of the source of information, whether research-based or anecdotal. For example, you may feel that it makes sense to you to improve your health by changing your diet from highly processed foods grown with pesticides and preserved with chemicals to organic foods cooked simply and served in balanced proportions in a serene environment. Or you may find it less risky to try a certain medication if a respected member of your support group has successfully taken it and you know that she has been having a set of symptoms very similar to your own.

Ideally, when making a treatment decision there's a relationship between the level of invasiveness of an approach and the weight of evidence of its safety and effectiveness. For example, because of the serious risks that accompany surgery to correct a Chiari malformation, before deciding to undergo it, you'd want to have a well-established database of evidence that the risks were worth taking. On the other hand, very low risk approaches—such as meditation—may be worth just giving a try.

It would be a mistake to assume that a healing approach is more risky simply because it's less conventional. For example, although the scenario of medication being offered by a family doctor is familiar and comfortable, the drug prescribed may carry a much greater risk of side effects than an aromatherapy treatment that seems "way out there" because it's relatively unfamiliar and practiced by an unlicensed person.

The following is a worksheet you can use to help you make treatment decisions. Because you'll probably consider several types of treatment, you may want to make copies of it.

WORKSHEET: FACTORS TO CONSIDER IN CHOOSING A TREATMENT

A. Circle the kinds of dysfunction you're trying to treat:

respiration and oxygenation

nutrition

digestion and metabolism

nerve transmission

immune response

repair of free radical damage

balance of subtle energies

circulation

detoxification

hormonal balance

structural/mechanical

sleep

emotional response

spiritual wellness

B. Rate each treatment you're considering according to the following criteria; circle the answer that is most true for you. When you've finished, compare your results to make treatment choices that will address all of your dysfunctions without inappropriate overlap. (The items marked with an "*" are answered in this book; the others are for you to think about or involve gathering information about your local resources.)

1. How many of these dysfunctions does the approach address? *

   All.

   Most.

   Just a few.

2. If this approach doesn't address all of your dysfunctions, are you willing to combine it with other approaches?

   Yes, whatever works.

   Yes, but I'd prefer a more streamlined approach.

   No.

3. Are there any incompatibilities between this approach and others that you are using or considering using?*

Yes. (What?)

No.

4. Is this approach available where you live?

Yes.

I'd need to travel, but I'm willing and able to do so.

No.

4. Can you afford this approach?

Yes.

It'll be a stretch.

No.

4. How safe or risky is this approach?*

Very safe.

There are some risks.

Very risky.

4. How much good research is there showing its effectiveness?*

A lot.

Some.

Not much.

4. How much reliable anecdotal evidence is there of its effectiveness?*

A lot.

Some.

Not much.

9. How long has this approach been around?*

More than 100 years.

Between 10 and 100 years.

It's brand new.

10. How well does the underlying philosophy of this approach fit with the way you think about your dysfunctions?

Perfect match.

Not really sure.

It doesn't seem right to me.

11. How well does the approach fit your personality and preferences in terms of the following criteria, on a scale from 1 to 5, with 5 being the best fit and 1 being the worst?

a. Being touched by a health professional.

1   2   3   4   5   N/A

b. Waiting a while for results.

1   2   3   4   5   N/A

c. Changing your diet.

1   2   3   4   5   N/A

d. Doing physical activity.

1   2   3   4   5   N/A

e. Taking medications.

1   2   3   4   5   N/A

f. Taking a lot of vitamins.

1   2   3   4   5   N/A

12. Do you feel capable of handling your own care—in terms of researching and carrying it out on your own—with this approach?

Yes, I'm ready.

Not so sure.

No way.

13. Are you aiming for symptom relief or for addressing the root of the problem?

Need relief ASAP.

I'm willing to wait for something that will last.

14. How weird does this approach feel to you?

Not weird at all.

It will be hard to get used to, but I'm up for it.

People will laugh at me or criticize me and I can't tolerate that.

How Long Will It Take to Work?

Once you decide on a treatment approach and begin applying it, there's a delicate balance to achieve between listening to your body—the best source of information on what works for you—and listening to other sources, like when your health practitioner tells you it may take a while for a treatment to begin to make a difference. For example, if you try a new kind of aerobic exercise, you'll probably know within twenty-four hours if it suits you. The same is true of some medications. However, it may take weeks to learn if a new nutritional supplement is making a difference. And with pharmaceuticals, although you may initially experience side effects that may make you believe the medication isn't good for you, if you wait a while the side effects may fade and the benefits kick in.

How to Choose a Practitioner

Let's return for a moment to the musical analogy from earlier in this chapter. In order to perform your symphony, you need musicians who both know how to play their instruments and are familiar with the piece of music you want to play. In other words, your health care providers must not only be masters of their own healing approaches, they must also have a deep knowledge of your FM or CFS, as well as any associated symptoms or additional syndromes you may be experiencing. This is equally true for holistic practitioners and mainstream health care providers.

In our health care marketplace, we have become accustomed to thinking of health care providers as authority figures whose advice we're supposed to follow without question; this is changing, in part due to the spread of alternative approaches. You may not realize that you're allowed to ask questions about a provider's credentials and experience before making an appointment—and that you can go into these matters in more depth during your first visit. You can also ask whether they've previously treated people with FM or CFS—and if so, how they conceptualize underlying causes and appropriate treatments.

Some health care providers may not like being questioned. Usually, this will be your first indicator that he or she isn't right for you. Other indicators may be explanations that are too simplistic or don't reflect recent knowledge of the field. What you want is a practitioner who gives explanations that you can understand, who answers your questions thoroughly and respectfully, and whom you feel good with. You need a practitioner with whom you can be a partner in your health care. After all, if you're going to conduct your symphony, you need musicians who will both give their best to the performance and take your direction as to how you want the piece of music performed.

To assess whether a practitioner has appropriate credentials, you need to know what kind of training is standard for a given approach. With MDs this is relatively easy because both training and licensing are standardized. Licensing not only assures an adequate level of training, it also typically indicates a reasonable level of ethical practice. Some other healing arts—including chiropractic, massage therapy, traditional Chinese medicine, and naturopathy—also have licensing procedures. However, licensure is a function of state government and varies from state to state. For example, right now naturopaths are only licensed in fourteen states, although other states are considering such laws. And although chiropractors are licensed in all fifty states, their permitted scope of practice varies quite a bit from state to state. Some of the healing arts aren't licensed in any state, so you'll need different ways of assessing practitioners' levels of training and expertise. We'll discuss the credentialing of practitioners in the chapters on the different healing arts.

Sometimes the best way to select a practitioner is to ask people you know and trust for referrals. If they can attest to the practitioner's experience with FM and CFS, collaborative attitude, and fair business practices, you'll know that you're in good hands.

Some Thoughts About Self-Care

The idea of independently taking care of ourselves can be very appealing. And with some of the alternative/complementary healing approaches, it's possible to do so. However, because the body is so complex—and healing methods are so well developed—it often makes more sense to work with a practitioner. Practitioners not only have training and experience, they often also have intuitive gifts for the kind of healing they do. When you simply read about healing methods on your own, you may be getting a simplified view of what the method is all about. You're also usually getting a one-size-fits-all approach when what you really want is a coherent plan tailored to your unique needs.

For all of these reasons, I believe the desire to self-heal is often best expressed in our daily actions—eating well, engaging in appropriate activity levels, managing stress, seeking spiritual sustenance, and carrying out the recommendations of our health care practitioner. These kinds of daily actions are powerful healing methods; we each need to become our own ultimate experts in these matters.

CHAPTER 4

Medical Treatments

This chapter will address treatment approaches for FM and CFS used primarily by MDs who aren't holistically oriented. The approaches described can be used to treat problems of respiration and oxygenation, digestion and metabolism, nerve transmission, immune response, circulation, hormonal balance, structural/mechanical alignment (specifically Chiari malformation), sleep and restoration, and emotional response.

Mainstream medicine has increasingly begun to incorporate alternative approaches into its treatment of complex chronic illnesses like FM and CFS. However, individual doctors will be at varying stages of their education regarding alternative approaches, ranging from those who have no knowledge of alternative approaches and use only the kinds of treatments detailed in this chapter, to those who practice integrative medicine, fully incorporating the best of both approaches—sometimes even avoiding the use of medications entirely. Those at the integrative end of the continuum are sometimes called naturopathic physicians or holistic MDs.

The treatment of FM and CFS by conventional medicine approaches usually involves four modalities: mild exercise, medication, the use of continuous positive airway pressure (CPAP) machines, and, for Chiari malformations, surgery.

Mild Exercise

People with FM and CFS are generally so tired and have such low energy that even the thought of exercise is overwhelming. Indeed, in people with FM or CFS too much exercise can lead to a worsening of symptoms, including a decrease in energy—not typical in healthy people, for whom exercise is generally energizing. However, if you stop exercising entirely, muscles may lose their conditioning and weaken. Thus, it can seem like you're damned if you do and damned if you don't.

The key to exercise for people with FM and CFS is to find the right level. Through trial and error, you can learn how to avoid both deconditioning and wearing yourself out. This has been referred to as the *Goldilocks Principle*, in honor of the famous character who found first a bowl of porridge that was too hot, then one that was too cold, and then finally, one that was just right. When you find a level of exercise that is just right, it can help you by decreasing depression, relieving pain, and increasing your strength, endurance, and range of motion.

When developing an exercise program for yourself, it's helpful to seek the advice of a personal trainer or physical therapist who is knowledgeable about working with people with FM and CFS. However, there's no surefire formula to follow; trial and error is needed to discover the exercise that is right for you. It's probably best to start very slowly, with a level of exercise that might not even seem like exercise. If it helps, think of it as movement rather than exercise. For instance, if you're in bed a lot of the day, just sitting up a little bit more might be a good start. Or, if you need to stay in bed or in a chair, you can rhythmically move whatever part of your body that you can move without pain. If you're able to be up and about, a good start might be walking a quarter of a block. But even that may be too much for some people. *You* are the expert on what your body can tolerate and thrive on. If you pay close attention to your body, you'll know when you've had enough exercise or if a certain kind of exercise isn't for you. It's important that you stop exercising before you're exhausted, so that it will be easier to rest and prepare for the next session.

Experiment with different types of exercise. Some people find that yoga or gentle martial arts—such as tai chi and qi gong—are more tolerable than other kinds of exercise. Swimming, underwater running, and exercising in waist-deep warm water are also helpful for some people.

Before increasing your exercise, assess how this first level is working out. When you've found an exercise type and level that you feel is helpful and not harmful, you can increase the level a tiny bit and assess again. The biggest mistake you can make is being too ambitious. For people with FM and CFS, a different, gentler standard is needed.

Medication

A wide array of medications are in use for FM and CFS. Although a few have been developed with FM and CFS in mind, and a few studies have been done on the effectiveness of specific drugs for people with FM and CFS, at this point, none have been approved by the FDA for use in FM or CFS. All of the medications listed here have previously been used with other illnesses or syndromes that share some specific symptoms with FM and CFS.

Using a medication for a purpose other than the one it was initially approved to treat is referred to as an *off-label use*. An example of off-label use is using baby aspirin to prevent second heart attacks. Typically there isn't much research on a medication's effectiveness for off-label uses. So, although general safety information is available for all prescription medicines, that information may or may not apply when the medication is used by people with FM or CFS. For safety information and for effectiveness in these off-label uses we must still rely, to a large degree, on anecdotal information.

With medications, the goal is usually symptom relief. For instance, a pain medication might relieve pain without addressing the ultimate cause of the pain—and as a result may need to be used indefinitely for continued pain management. When medications are used for a long time, adverse effects can accumulate and medications may stop being as effective as they once were.

One issue that arises with medication use in people with FM and CFS is drug hypersensitivity. Just as you may be extra sensitive to other things that most people take in stride, so you may be more sensitive to a medication. Thus, you may require a much lower dose than standard. Some physicians are unaware of this need to begin with a lower dose; as a result, a medication may be discontinued due to side effects that wouldn't have occurred at the proper individualized dose and, therefore, the medication's potential benefits may be missed. Even without this hypersensitivity, though, finding the right medication usually takes some trial and error.

Another issue with medications for FM and CFS is that, quite often, medications are used in combinations. This may be done to increase their effectiveness in treating a certain symptom, or to treat multiple symptoms. There's a lot of information available about the dangers of interactions between specific pairs of medications. However, once you get beyond two or three medications, it's much harder to predict the effects of combining them. It's also important to be aware that some herbs and other nutritional supplements interact with medications in dangerous ways. There are a number of books and Web sites that detail these interactions, such as the *Physicians' Desk Reference (PDR) for Herbal Medicines* (Medical Economics, Gruenwald, and PDR staff 2004).

The following is a listing of many of the medications in use for FM and CFS and associated symptoms. Where possible, both the generic name and the trade name are listed, with trade names in parentheses and capitalized. Because new research is being done all of the time—and because there are important safety issues involved—it's important to always check for the latest information before beginning a new medication. The Web sites for the Centers for Disease Control and the National Institutes of Health are good sources of information about medications for FM and CFS—they're updated as new research emerges. Also, each medication usually has its own official Web page where you can find a lot of information about the drug, including its side effects. *Every* medication has side effects, some more serious than others. It's critically important that you learn about these side effects and make your decision about whether or not to take a given medication carefully. (The medications that have been shown to have beneficial effects for FM and CFS patients, either in research studies or extended clinical usage, are marked with an "*"; those with particularly strong research backing are marked "**".)

Painkillers

There are a number of approaches to relieving the pain of FM and CFS, including both prescription and over-the-counter medicines.

Nonsteroidal Anti-Inflammatory Drugs (NSAIDS)

NSAIDs are used for pain in FM and CFS, even when the pain isn't directly associated with inflammation.

- Available over the counter: naproxen (Aleve, Anaprox, Naprosyn), *ibuprofen (Advil, Bayer Select, Motrin, Nuprin), *acetaminophen (Tylenol, Datril, Excedrin)

- By prescription: celecoxib (Celebrex), **tramadol hydro-chloride (Ultram, Ultracet—with added acetaminophen), piroxicam (Feldene), nabumetone (Relafen)

Opioids (Narcotics)

Opioids work by either blocking or altering pain messages sent to the brain by the nerves. Opioids have been found only minimally effective in relieving pain in FM, possibly because the body's internal pain relief systems are already maximized and can't be increased with external opioids. Because of opioids' highly addictive nature, most people prefer to find other methods of pain control. Opioids also carry a risk of an increase in pain.

- morphine sulfate (Duramorph), hydrocodone (Vicodin), oxycodone (Percodan, Percocet, Roxicodone, OxyContin), methadone

Topical Analgesics

Topical analgesics are medicated lotions that can be applied externally to areas of pain.

- capsaicin (Zostrix)—an ointment made from the purified form of the active ingredient in chili peppers; it relieves pain by tiring the pain receptors in the region of the pain, so the receptors can no longer communicate the pain sensation for a period of time

- *024 Fibromyalgia (Swiss Medica)—a topical analgesic made from camphor and other botanical oils

Anesthetics

Anesthetics are sometimes injected into trigger points or infused into veins to numb pain.

- *lidocaine, procaine; lidocaine is also now available in the form of a patch (Lidoderm) that adheres to the skin over the area of pain

Muscle Relaxers

Muscle relaxers are used for general pain relief and muscle spasms.

- **cyclobenzaprine (Flexeril), *tizanidine (Zanaflex), orphenadrine citrate (Norflex), metaxalone (Skelaxin), methocarbamol (Robaxin), **carisoprodol (Soma)

Antidepressants

Tricyclics

Low doses of these antidepressants are used for sleep problems and pain in people with FM and CFS. This class of medications also has antiallergy effects.

- doxepin (Adapin, Sinequan), **amitriptyline (Elavil, Etrafon, Limbitrol, Triavil), desipramine (Norpramin), *nortriptyline (Pamelor, Aventyl)

MAO Inhibitors

This category of medications is rarely prescribed, because its potential for severe interaction effects requires important restrictions on the consumption of certain foods, drugs, and supplements for those taking them.

- *selegiline (Emsam, Carbex)—a new MAO inhibitor delivered through a skin patch, just approved by the FDA; it has the advantage of bypassing the need for strict dietary restrictions, at least at low doses

- *moclobemide (Manerix)—not available in the U.S.

Selective Serotonin Reuptake Inhibitors (SSRIs)

New research indicates a possible effect of these medications on the immune system, as well as on pain and depression (O'Connell et al. 2006).

- *fluoxetine (Prozac), *sertraline (Zoloft), citalopram (Celexa), escitalopram (Lexapro), paroxetine (Paxil)

Atypical Antidepressants

This class of medications, also called multiple reuptake inhibitors, optimizes availability of more than one neurotransmitter.

- *trazodone (Desyrel), *venlafaxine (Effexor), *nefazodone (Serzone), **duloxetine hydrochloride (Cymbalta), bupropion (Wellbutrin), mirtazapine (Remeron), **milnacipran (Ixel), *reboxetine (Edronax)

Antianxiety Medications

For Insomnia

- alprazolam (Xanax), *lorazepam (Ativan), diazepam (Valium)

For Neurological Symptoms

This medication is used for physical symptoms due to nervous system problems such as vertigo, burning or tenderness of the skin, and nervous limb movements.

- *clonazepam (Klonopin)

Sleep Aids

Sedative Hypnotics

- *zolpidem (Ambien), triazolam (Halcion), *eszopiclone (Lunesta), temazepam (Restoril)
- zaleplon (Sonata)

Noncontrolled Sleep Medicines

This medication has a different mechanism of action than the ones listed above; it's said to be less addictive than other sleep medications.

■ ramelteon (Rozerem)

Stimulants

This medication is used in cases of narcolepsy or excessive daytime sleepiness, as identified by a sleep study.

■ modafinil (Provigil)

Antimicrobials

These medications are used only if a specific infectious agent is found; the use of these medications in people with FM and CFS is relatively rare and highly controversial.

Antibiotics

■ doxycycline (Vibramycin), azithromycin (Zithromax), ciprofloxacin (Cipro), neomycin (used by a few doctors in the treatment of irritable bowel syndrome)

Antifungals

■ *fluconazole (Diflucan)—tablets; *nystatin (Biostatin, Nilstat)—vaginal cream or tablets

Antivirals

■ acyclovir (Zovirax), famciclovir (Famvir), valganciclovir (Valcyte)

Antiparasitics

- metronidazole (Flagyl), iodoquinol (Yodoxin)

Immune Enhancers

These medications work to strengthen the immune system itself.

- *isoprinosine (Imunovir)—has both immune enhancing and antiviral properties

- (*Ampligen)—used to stimulate the production of *interferons*, a family of immune response modifiers known to have antiviral activity

- (*sizofiran)—an immunostimulant extracted from suehirotake mushrooms; it's currently in phase II trials for the treatment of CFS

- gammaglobulin—pooled human immune globulin; it contains antibody molecules directed against a broad range of common infectious agents

- staphylococcus toxoid and mycobacterium vaccines—killed organisms prepared and administered as vaccines, in an attempt to stimulate a specific immune response

Thyroid Medications

This group of medications is used to strengthen the function of the thyroid gland.

- levothyroxine (Synthroid, Levothroid, Levoxyl, Unithroid), liothyronine (Cytomel)

- *natural thyroid (Armour Thyroid, Westhroid, Naturethroid)—made of dried thyroid gland of pigs; it's used only rarely by physicians without a holistic orientation

Antiseizure Medications

These medications are used for sleep and pain in FM and CFS patients.

■ *gabapentin (Neurontin), **pregabalin (Lyrica)

Antiallergy Medications

Nonsedating Antihistamines

■ desloratadine (Clarinex), fexofenadine (Allegra), cetirizine (Zyrtec)

Sedating Antihistamines

This medication is used primarily for its side effect of inducing sleep.

■ diphenhydramine (Benadryl)

Antihypotensive/Antitachycardia Medications

These medications are used for patients with positive tilt table tests.

■ *fludrocortisone (Florinef)

■ beta-blockers—e.g., atenolol (Tenormin)

■ *midodrine (ProAmatine)—directly increases blood pressure

■ desmopressin—a hormone that decreases urination

Anti-Parkinsonian Medications

These drugs increase the availability of the neurotransmitter dopamine and are used in FM and CFS for restless limb syndrome and periodic leg movements of sleep. It should be noted that the use of these medications can trigger the onset of restless leg symptoms earlier in the day.

- levodopa (Sinemet, Larodopa, Atamet), *pergolide (Per-max), *pramipexole (Mirapex), *ropinirole (Requip)

Cough Suppressants

The use of these medications for FM and CFS is controversial and represents a fairly large and creative departure from the use for which the medications were intended and approved.

- guaifenesin—used to lessen excessive accumulation of phosphate and calcium in the body tissues; pioneered by R. Paul St. Amand

- dextromethorphan—an ingredient in cough medicine; because it lowers the threshold for the coughing reflex, it may also lower sensitivity to pain

Irritable Bowel Treatments

These medicines are used for diarrhea, constipation, and other bowel symptoms.

- tegaserod (Zelnorm) for constipation-dominant IBS, alosetron (Lotronex) for diarrhea-dominant IBS

- pinaverium (Dicetel), hyoscine (Buscopan)

Corticosteroids

Mineralcorticoids

- *fludrocortisone (Florinef)

Glucocorticoids

- *hydrocortisone (Hydrocortone, Cortef)—has anti-inflammatory effects and may help with symptoms of adrenal fatigue

Anticoagulants

This medication is used to address excessive coagulation of the blood.

- heparin (Calciparine, Liquaemin)

Anticataplexy, Antinarcolepsy Medications

This medication is used for altered sleep patterns; it's said to increase deep stages of sleep and growth hormone secretion. It carries some very serious side effects.

- **sodium oxybate (Xyrem)—a highly controlled substance due to its potential for abuse

Acetylcholinesterase Inhibitors

The medications in this class increase the availability of the neurotransmitter *acetylcholine*, which can lead to improved memory and cognition.

- galantamine (Razadyne)—usually used in Alzheimer's disease

- *pyridostigmine (Mestinon)—similar to galantamine; some research has shown that pyridostigmine increases release of growth hormone in people with FM and CFS

Serotonin Receptor Medications

Because levels of the neurotransmitter serotonin are high in some people with FM and CFS, and low in others, new medications are being tried that affect availability of serotonin in various targeted ways, in order to reduce pain.

- tropisetron (Navoban), *pindolol (Visken)

Continuous Positive Airway Pressure (CPAP) Machine

Among other sleep disorders, many people with FM and CFS suffer from sleep apnea. In sleep apnea, breathing may briefly stop hundreds of times every night. When breathing stops, the body then rouses itself enough to restore normal breathing; this leads to shallow, disrupted sleep—and extreme fatigue during the day. A leading treatment for sleep apnea is the use of a CPAP machine; CPAP machines blow air into the airways through a mask worn over the mouth and nose. This continuous air pressure doesn't substitute for your own breathing; instead, it encourages the airways to stay open to allow normal breathing to continue.

Sleep apnea should be assessed with an overnight sleep study. If the study shows that you have sleep apnea, you may be asked to try out a CPAP machine that very same night to see if it works for you. If you do have sleep apnea, your doctor or a sleep specialist can help you decide if CPAP is the best approach to treating it.

Surgery for Chiari Malformation

In chapter 2 we discussed Chiari malformation, a condition in which the lower part of the brain extends down into the upper portion of the spinal column, creating a constriction. This constriction can then result in many of the same symptoms seen in FM and CFS. Some people find that surgical interventions help them achieve symptom relief; this isn't, however, applicable to the vast majority of people with FM and CFS. Your physician can guide you through assessing this and deciding whether surgery is indicated; obviously, this surgery isn't a treatment to be taken lightly.

CHAPTER 5

Nutritional Approaches I: Food

Maximizing nutritional intake can affect every aspect of health. People with FM and CFS seem to be more prone to being adversely affected by food than other people and often start to feel better when their diet changes. It may be that unhealthy foods are a direct cause of symptoms or it may be that when other body systems are compromised, the body is less able to tolerate foods that don't support health. Either way, modifying what you eat is a significant treatment option for people with FM and CFS. Although diet changes may be challenging to make, they also allow you to take action several times a day to improve your health. This can be a boon for people with FM and CFS, who often feel that their health is out of their control.

The "Sad" Standard American Diet

By now most Americans know that many of the foods they eat aren't good for them, but still manage to ignore this fact when it comes to their daily eating. People who speak of the harm caused by the modern American diet are often dismissed as alarmists or worse. But there's a lot of evidence that they're right. Because we're accustomed to the foods we eat and can't easily envision a pleasurable life without them, it can be difficult to allow ourselves to take this information in. And yet, few people would dispute the idea that feeling good is pleasurable and feeling ill is not. Most of us can easily call upon anecdotal examples that support unhealthy diets—Uncle So-and-So, who ate pork every day of his life and lived to a ripe old age; or Grandma, who lived on candy and was still vigorous and strong when she died at 101. But these are exceptions rather than the rule; the rule is not a pretty picture.

Some experts estimate that as much as 70 percent of illness in America is caused by lifestyle factors—e.g., what we eat, how much we move, and how we handle our stress. Making good food choices is an option that very few Americans take advantage of. The standard diet in most developed nations is so far removed from healthy eating that many people don't even know how to consistently eat food that's good for them. It's hard to buy healthy food in stores and restaurants and most people lack information on what foods are healthy and how to prepare them. Reports in the media, side by side with advertisements for food products, further confuse matters.

How Do You Sort Out What's True About Healthy Eating?

In recent years there's been a lot of talk about one or the other *macronutrients*—basic building blocks of all food: proteins, carbohydrates, and fats—being bad for you. The proponents for these restrictions all make convincing arguments. When you look at the science, one thing that's clear is that whatever food you eat, quality matters. It's now accepted that there are good fats—e.g., olive oil—and bad fats—e.g., trans fats, chemically transformed from liquids into semi-solids. Good fats are essential to your health, and bad ones are harmful. We've known for a long time that whole grains and other complex carbohydrates—such as those found in beans—are better for you than simple carbohydrates like table sugar. Similarly, protein foods are better for you when they're free of harmful chemicals like the mercury found in some fish, the heterocyclic amines (HCAs) found in meats grilled over high heat, and the antibiotics fed to chickens. In these dialogues about low carbohydrate or low fat diets, issues have become confused through ignoring the more important issue: the quality of the food itself.

One likely reason different studies have found carbohydrates and fats to be bad for you is probably because the healthy and unhealthy versions of these foods were examined together—muddying the results of the research. Similarly, low fat and low carbohydrate diets may work well for people simply because while on the diet they pay better attention to what they eat, and in the process eliminate some of the more unhealthy foods. These diets generally cause people to eat more vegetables, and in some cases more fruit as well. This is a basic food guideline that nearly every nutrition expert agrees on, both as a method of weight management and as a way of providing maximum nourishment for our bodies.

Much of eating healthily is common sense, but you may not know how to implement it—not surprising given the world we live in. And when you're already feeling tired and sick, it can be overwhelming to try to figure it all out.

A Healthy Diet

The following are some simple guidelines in choosing foods to support your health:

Eat Food in a Form Close to Its Most Natural State

The more processed a food is, the more of its nutritional value is lost. For example, an unpeeled apple is better than applesauce—which is better than apple juice. The reason the food's natural state is better is that it contains the whole package of nutrients and supporting factors that help you derive the most benefit from it. For example, the whole apple has fiber, which will allow you to digest the sugars in the apple in a slower, more balanced way.

Choose Foods Grown Without the Use of Pesticides and Herbicides

When you eat food grown with pesticides and herbicides, you may be consuming poisons along with your food—and to some degree, negating the food's ability to keep you healthy. Processing these toxins taxes your body's ability to deal with other, less avoidable dangers.

Avoid Foods That Have Harmful or Addictive Effects

Refined sugar has a number of adverse effects on human health, including suppression of the immune system (Appleton 1996). Paul Cheney, a leading expert on FM and CFS, believes that people with FM and CFS are particularly vulnerable to the adverse effects of sugar because their bodies can't break it down properly (Sieverling 2005). This results in excess lactic acid in the bloodstream, symptoms of which may be muscle pain, headaches, and psychological symptoms such as panic attacks (Feinstein 1998). Keep in mind, though, that artificial sweeteners aren't the answer as there are serious questions about their safety.

It's also important to avoid caffeine; caffeine can interfere with sleep and alter cardiac function, among other effects. Some people believe that it may also block mineral absorption (Feinstein 1998). Alcohol can also interfere with such things as cardiac function, body temperature regulation, and liver function. Both of these substances are addictive and tax the liver's ability to detoxify the body.

Prepare Foods to Make Them More Digestible

Lightly steaming some vegetables—such as broccoli—can make nutrients more accessible, and help you eat more of them. On the other hand, heating some foods to very high temperatures—particularly oils— can make them not only less nutritious, but may also turn them into health risks. Many believe that eating foods raw makes sense because the enzymes in the food that are needed to digest it thus remain viable. It's not clear what balance of raw versus cooked foods is appropriate for a given individual, but it's a factor to consider.

Eat Fresh Foods

If food has been around for too long, it's either past its prime—in which case much of the nutritional value is gone; spoiled—obviously not good for you; or preserved with chemicals toxic not only to the organisms that would have made the food spoil, but also to our bodies.

Consume Food in Appropriate Amounts and Proportions

If we eat either too much or not enough food, our bodies won't be at their best. We probably all differ in the proportions of the macronutrients that are best for us, but if one or more of these is consumed to excess, it's likely to contribute to health problems. For example, eating too much protein can stress the kidneys.

Finding Your Optimal Diet

So, how do you translate these guidelines into a menu plan that fits with your body, your budget, and your energy level? First, there isn't any one diet that's ideal for everybody. It may be that your optimal diet is vegetarian, vegan, raw foods, or macrobiotic. It may be that including fish, chicken, and other meat is best for you. The main criteria of a good diet are that it includes all of your macronutrients in whatever proportions work best for you and that it makes you feel good over the long term. Above all, it's important to eat only real food, rather than preservatives, pesticides, artificial coloring and flavoring agents, bleaches, and other additives.

In the first century BC, the philosopher Lucretius said, "What is food to one man may be fierce poison to others." This still makes sense. Some people live on a diet dominated by foods like dairy, citrus, and wheat; others will be made ill by the very same foods. This is particularly true of people with FM and CFS, because of the high incidence of food sensitivities and digestive problems. Some people thrive on raw foods; others literally can't stomach them. Some people eat their largest meal in the evening; others need to graze throughout the day. Each person is unique and needs his or her own special diet.

Sometimes you'll need different foods—and different quantities of food—than at other times, based on overall health, level of activity, the seasons, or other factors. By listening to your body you'll know which foods to eat and how much. Offer your body clean whole foods prepared in a way that maximizes their nutritional value, and then take note of how you feel. The foods that make you feel good not just while you're eating them, but also twenty minutes, two hours, or two days later, are the ones that are probably your best fuel.

One way to discover your best fuels is through an elimination diet. This involves removing one food at a time from your diet for a period of about two weeks and making careful observations of how you feel. Keep a diary of what you eat, when you eat it, and what changes you observe in your symptoms—this will make it easier to find patterns. It usually makes sense to start with the foods you're accustomed to eating most often, since there is a tendency to develop sensitivities to foods that are consumed frequently. If eliminating a food has no effect, try removing other foods from your diet one at a time for a period of two weeks, until you discover your optimal foods.

The Logistics of Eating Well

Unless you have a health food store with a high quality take-out deli and can afford to let them prepare your food, eating health-supportive foods on a regular basis will probably involve cooking. Any number of excellent cookbooks can help you learn how to select and prepare foods that meet the criteria laid out in this chapter. However, cookbooks tend to focus on complex recipes—what I call "company food"—which can seem overwhelming on days when it may be exhausting or painful simply to get to the kitchen, let alone tackle a difficult, multistep recipe. For everyday foods, it's often best to eat more simply. What a lot of people don't realize is that simple foods—like vegetables, whole grains, and simple protein foods—are very easy to prepare and can taste delicious.

One way to plan meals that are quick, easy, and good for you is to consider the vegetables (one or more) as the center of the meal and then add accessories to them, just as you might add a scarf and belt to a simple black dress. In the case of food, accessories are protein foods (meat, fish, beans, tofu, nuts, seeds, etc.) and whole grains (rice, quinoa, couscous, bread, etc). Then, just as you might add earrings to your outfit to finish it off, you can add a sauce or a condiment to the meal to increase its appeal. For example, if you have broccoli you can lightly steam it, and serve it dressed in olive oil and lemon juice on a bed of brown jasmine rice, with grilled chicken on the side. Or you could sauté it in garlic, add cannellini beans, and serve it over whole grain pasta with or without prepared tomato sauce, olives, or cheese. Or you could use it in a salad with mixed greens and other vegetables as a side dish with a tofu burger on whole grain bread. Of course, you should adjust your menu to your needs, avoiding whatever foods don't make you feel good. You just need some basic cooking techniques and a selection of ingredients—then you can use your imagination to accessorize your vegetables in a way that suits your tastes, nutritional needs, and energy level.

If your energy tends to be limited, you can cook larger batches of foods at a time of the day or week when you're feeling a little better—or if you're lucky, maybe a friend will do it for you—and then have extra for several days worth of easy meals. Soups are particularly conducive to this. Provided you're careful to avoid unsafe ingredients, another option is to buy some items already prepared. For instance, canned beans are generally available with little or no added ingredients and are still pretty nutritious. Roasted chicken from the prepared foods section of a supermarket or deli might be another good choice, and can provide a variety of meals; veggie burgers just need to be warmed up. Another great shortcut is packages of prewashed organic salad greens, now available in most supermarkets. If you develop a repertoire of one or two weeks worth of meals, you can eliminate the problem of having to figure out what to eat for any given meal, and still have variety.

It's Not Just What You Eat, It's How You Eat It

Another important element of eating in a health-supportive manner is to eat in a peaceful environment and in a relaxed state of mind. When your body is on alert, preparing to face real or perceived danger, it isn't ready to properly digest food. Food should be eaten slowly, chewed well, and savored. When we eat in a hurry, we miss out on the first stage of digestion that takes place in the mouth and we deprive ourselves of one of the great pleasures in life: enjoying our meals and being nourished by them to a state of vibrant health.

CHAPTER 6

Nutritional Approaches II: Supplements

The majority of nonpharmaceutical treatment approaches now being used for FM and CFS involve courses of specific nutritional supplements, intended to address specific imbalances in the body. Dozens of substances are being used this way—the tricky part is knowing which ones to try. In chapter 2 we talked about the kinds of things that go wrong in the bodies of people with FM and CFS and how to assess them. Use this information as a basis for making decisions about whether to try any of the nutritional supplements. If you know the underlying cause of your symptoms, you can read this chapter with an eye toward which supplements will address that cause. Supplements can be used to address all of the elements of health.

Although it would be ideal for everybody to get all of the nutrition they need from food, in many cases this simply isn't realistic. People with FM and CFS tend to be deficient—or marginally deficient—in a number of nutrients. It's believed this is due to problems with utilizing nutrients rather than to a failure to eat properly.

Can You Do This On Your Own?

Many people choose nutritional supplements based on reading about them or hearing about them from other sources, and then decide on their own what dosage to take. This is one of the strengths of this kind of approach—it empowers you to take charge of your own health. But each of our bodies is unique; just because one person benefits from taking a certain supplement for a specific condition doesn't mean another person with the same condition will find that supplement equally effective—or even tolerable. As with food, you can have a sensitivity to certain supplement products due to their ingredients or preparation methods. You may also simply have a better response to one approach than another.

It's helpful to have a health care professional guide you. Health professionals can also order tests that will give you specific information about your body's biochemistry. However, available tests aren't always reliable ways of determining real nutritional needs (Werbach 2000). Some practitioners recommend hair analyses as a reasonably priced way to assess mineral status. Applied kinesiology is an approach that's quite effective not only in determining which supplements you need, but which forms of them your body best responds to (see chapter 8).

Here are some things to keep in mind as you work out a treatment plan:

Supplements Are Supplemental

Supplements are meant to be *supplemental* sources of nutrition—not primary sources. Before investing time and money in supplements, first pursue dietary changes to maximize the nutritional value of your food.

Supplements Are Powerful

Some nutritional supplements can cause harm if used incorrectly. Unfortunately, supplement manufacturers generally don't provide any warnings like those that pharmaceutical companies are required to provide. For some of the better known supplements this isn't a problem— for instance, guidelines can readily be found for how much of a given vitamin or mineral to use. But for less well-known supplements, standards may not have been established yet and not much experience may have accumulated—making it much harder to search out the information you need.

Another related issue is that standard dosages aren't the same as therapeutic dosages. Standard dosages are based on what is normal for healthy people, not sick people. And recommended daily dosages are averages, rather than information about your own personal nutritional needs, which vary quite a bit from person to person. Also, some prescription drugs deplete minerals; this will affect your supplement needs, as will your dietary intake of nutrients and other factors. People with a much higher need for a given supplement can get averaged out with people who have a much lower need—yielding a dosage that's right for neither.

Supplements Are Profitable

Nutritional supplements are sold by companies that operate for profit. It's in their best interest for you to believe in the value of their products. Although this is true of most consumer products—including pharmaceuticals—with nutritional supplements, the profit motive is combined with a lack of external quality standards and the fact that supplements can have potent health effects. This combination carries with it the risks that you may waste your money on products that don't do what their manufacturers say they will, and that you may suffer actual harm.

As with any kind of business, the owners and managers of companies producing supplements vary quite a bit in terms of their ethics and integrity. Just as it's better to buy a major appliance from a manufacturer that has stood the test of time and is well-known for good service and fair business practices, so it's better to purchase supplements from companies that are known for putting quality above profits—or that earn their profits from selling high quality products rather than large amounts of poorer quality products. With supplements it can be hard to discern which companies to trust. And if the quality of the supplement is poor, it will be difficult to tease out any direct effect it has on your health.

So how can you be certain about a supplement's quality? One thing you can do is visit www.consumerlab.com. There, for a reasonably priced subscription fee, you can access the results of tests of many brands of a wide variety of nutrients. You can also visit the Web sites of the companies that make the supplements you're considering and read what they say about their manufacturing processes. Those that go to great lengths to ensure the quality of their products will be proud to tell you about what they do.

Another way to assess the quality of supplements is price. Although not all high-priced supplements are of high quality, it's usually true that products priced much lower than their competitors are of inferior quality; it's expensive to produce really high quality supplements.

It's also a good idea to get recommendations from trusted health professionals regarding which brands to use. The best supplements generally aren't available in drug stores, supermarkets, or health food stores. Because of concerns that supplements would be used unsafely if available to the general public, some of the better companies only sell products through health care practitioners. Of course, there are some notable exceptions to this. Also, it may seem that selling products creates a conflict of interest for reputable holistic health care professionals—since they'll reap profits from the sales, they'll have a strong incentive to prescribe them. Although this is probably true of some practitioners, in my experience the majority sell supplements in their offices simply to give you access to the best ones. Moreover, the products that are sold this way are subject to the close scrutiny of the practitioners selling them—who will usually also have better resources for evaluating them.

Quality of Supplements

The following are some of the issues involved in the quality of supplements. It may seem overwhelming to have to think about all of these issues; generally, if you stick with the best brands—as described above—all or most of these issues will be addressed by the manufacturer.

How pure the product is. Some products have material added to them, either to keep costs low, keep the product fresh, or discourage clumping. Also, chemical solvents may be used in the preparation of the product, leaving a residue behind. These additional ingredients may or may not be harmful.

The concentration of active ingredients. Some supplements are sold in doses so small that they aren't effective unless you take a lot of them—which can then make their cost prohibitive.

Whether products are natural or synthetic. Vitamins created in the lab tend to have a longer shelf life, provide a more consistent dosage, and be both less expensive and easier to handle. However, although a synthetic product's chemical composition may be technically identical to the natural form's, many people believe that our bodies don't use synthetic products exactly as they use natural ones. In some cases, a synthesized form may not work as well when it's taken in isolation, without the other natural substances or cofactors that help the body make best use of it. For example, although ascorbic acid—the main component of vitamin

C—can be synthesized with a chemical composition identical to the vitamin C derived from natural sources such as rose hips and acerola cherries, without the supporting natural substances called bioflavonoids, the synthetic ascorbic acid isn't as useful. A further problem is that the term "natural" can mean many different things and encompasses ingredients that aren't the best sources of a given nutrient.

The form in which the supplement is supplied. In some cases, a tablet won't dissolve well enough to fully deliver a supplement to your body; a capsule may be preferable. Similarly, sometimes a liquid will be the form that allows maximum utilization of the supplement, but other forms will be sold as well.

Some Cautions and Disclaimers

The fact that supplements are available without a prescription doesn't mean they aren't powerful. Nutrients found in supplements are generally much more concentrated than those found in foods and can affect many bodily functions. For example, sometimes the use of a supplement will actually cause the body to make less of the same substance, resulting in the opposite of the desired effect. And, too, sometimes changing the amount of one substance alters the delicate balance between that substance and another in your body, causing additional symptoms. Moreover, some nutrients are depleted during the utilization of others.

I'm not a physician and cannot prescribe supplements. Even physicians should never prescribe supplements for somebody they've never met or examined. Choose a health care practitioner who will work with you to develop a treatment plan. What follows is intended as a guide to help you decide which supplements you may want to learn more about. I'm focusing here on supplements commonly used in treating FM and CFS for which there is some substantiating research available. There are rapid developments in this area, though, so you may want to subscribe to one of the reputable FM/CFS newsletters to stay abreast of new research (for example, the ones published by immunesupport.com and fmaware.org).

There are also many good resources for further information about nutrients, such as *Staying Healthy with Nutrition* by Elson Haas; *Earl Mindell's New Vitamin Bible*; *Understanding Nutrition* by Eleanor Noss Whitney, Sharon Rady Rolfs, and Ellie Whitney; and the Web site of the Office of Dietary Supplements (ods.od.nih.gov). Please consult experts and proceed with caution.

Fat-Soluble Vitamins

Vitamin A: Vitamin A is actually a group of related vitamins involved in vision, cell differentiation, production of antibodies, reproduction, and the integrity of the skin and mucous membranes. It can be helpful in healing the gut and optimizing immune function. Vitamin A deficiencies are rare, but can sometimes be seen in people suffering from malabsorption of fat, due to irritations of the intestines—as is often seen with FM and CFS. Vitamin A is best known to the FM and CFS community for its antioxidant properties. However, unlike vitamin C, which is a water-soluble vitamin with antioxidant properties, excess intake of vitamin A can be a problem. Sometimes it can be helpful to take *carotenoids*—like beta-carotene, lutein, and lycopene—which are precursors to vitamin A and can be taken in higher dosages without the risk of toxicity. Carotenoids are pigments that produce the orange and red colors in some vegetables. Some carotenoids also have additional antioxidant properties.

Vitamin D: Vitamin D is both found in food and can be synthesized by our bodies from sunlight. Vitamin D is involved in regulating mineral balance in the body, specifically calcium and phosphorus to promote bone density. It's also involved in regulation of the immune system and cell growth and differentiation. Vitamin D deficiency is a common cause of musculoskeletal pain. People who have difficulty digesting fat, people with dark skin, people who avoid the sun and always use sunscreen, and people who drink a lot of coffee may be at risk for vitamin D deficiency (NIH Office of Dietary Supplements 2005). Vitamin D deficiency is very common; your doctor can order a test to check your levels. I've found no studies that specifically address vitamin D supplementation in FM and CFS, but Sullivan (2004) details many of the latest findings on vitamin D—one of which is that vitamin D deficiency is sometimes mistaken for FM or CFS.

Vitamin E: There are eight forms of vitamin E; gamma tocopherol is the most active form. Vitamin E protects the body from oxidative damage, supports the immune system, and assists in the breakdown of some fats. Vitamin E can be deficient in people who have difficulty digesting fats, as can be the case with irritable bowel syndrome. One early study (Steinberg 1942) showed a beneficial effect of vitamin E supplementation in people with FM, but there hasn't been much follow-up research so far. Anecdotal evidence also suggests that vitamin E may help with restless leg syndrome.

Water-Soluble Vitamins

B-complex vitamins: This category includes thiamin (B_1), riboflavin (B_2), niacin (B_3), pantothenic acid (B_5), pyridoxine (B_6), biotin (B_7), folate, and B_{12}. These vitamins are involved in nearly every function of the body including energy production, and can be depleted by chronic stress. Supplementation supports the adrenal glands, which are involved in the stress response. B vitamins have been found to be deficient in people with CFS (Heap, Peters, and Wessely 1999).

> **Thiamin:** Thiamin is needed for nerve and muscle function and deriving energy from food. Eisinger (1998) notes that the symptoms of thiamin deficiency parallel those of FM, and proposes thiamin supplementation for pain relief as well as normalization of neurotransmitter function. Multiple studies have found that increases in thiamin availability have led to improvements in mood (Benton and Donohoe 1999).
>
> **Nicotinamide adenine dinucleotide hydrogen (NADH):** NADH is synthesized in the body from niacin. An antioxidant, it also stimulates the production of ATP and helps with neurotransmitter function. A randomized double-blind study by Forsyth et al. (1999) showed a positive effect on energy production with NADH supplementation in people with CFS.
>
> **Vitamin B_5:** Vitamin B_5, also called pantothenic acid, is required for the digestion of fats and carbohydrates and is used in the production of antibodies; because it also plays a role in the production of adrenal hormones, it can be helpful for people with FM and CFS who need adrenal support.
>
> **Vitamin B_6:** Vitamin B_6 is involved in metabolizing protein, converting tryptophan into serotonin, and red blood cell formation. It's also active in the immune and nervous systems. Vitamin B_6 is thought to affect cognition, but one rigorous review of the literature found supplementation had no substantial effect on cognition (Malouf and Grimley 2003).
>
> **Folate (folic acid):** Folate is needed for tissue growth, cell function, and protein synthesis. Jacobson et al. (1993) found lower folate levels in half of their small sample of people with CFS. Although Kaslow, Rucker, and Onishi (1989) found no benefit from folate supplementation in people with CFS, Werbach (2000) argues that

their dosage wasn't high enough and their study didn't run long enough to have a positive effect.

Vitamin B$_{12}$: Vitamin B$_{12}$ is involved in nerve function, formation of red blood cells, and regulation of homocysteine. Low levels are associated with neuropathy and fatigue. Because high doses appear to be necessary in some people—particularly the elderly, who may have trouble absorbing oral doses—B$_{12}$ is sometimes injected as well as taken orally. B$_{12}$ is sometimes administered even if vitamin levels in blood tests are normal, because these tests don't always offer accurate measurements of B$_{12}$ in the body (Werbach 2000). In Werbach's review of the literature on B$_{12}$ supplementation (2000), he notes that although there are no high quality studies affirming its value in people with FM and CFS, studies with other patient groups indicate that it may be effective in relieving pain and fatigue and increasing well-being. It can be taken with B$_6$ and folate to maintain balance among these B vitamins.

Vitamin C: In addition to improving immune function, vitamin C is also involved in the synthesis of collagen and norepinephrine. Vitamin C deficiencies have been found to be related to depression, pain, fatigue, and capillary fragility. Research in other patient populations with similar symptoms suggests vitamin C supplementation could be helpful for people with FM and CFS (Werbach 2000). Kodama, Kodama, and Murakami (1996) found an intravenous infusion of a combination of two forms of vitamin C beneficial in people with CFS, and vitamin C supplementation has been recommended for people with low cysteine levels. Vitamin C is better absorbed when taken with bioflavonoids (Vinson and Bose 1988).

Co Q 10: An antioxidant also known as vitamin Q or ubiquinone, Co Q 10 assists in energy production and helps the heart pump. A controlled clinical study of Co Q 10 in people with postexertional fatigue by Judy showed impressive increases in exercise tolerance (Werbach 2000). Many medications, including the cholesterol-lowering statins, cause lower levels of Co Q 10.

Flavonoids or bioflavonoids: Because of the many different ways flavonoids—including rutin, hesperidin, lycopene, quercetin, and genistein—act in the body, this group of nutrients defies categorization. Flavonoids are often broken down into subcategories such as isoflavones, anthocyanidins, flavans, flavonols, flavones, and flavanones. They're found in the pigments of fruits, vegetables, and soy as well as those in beverages such as tea, wine, and beer. Best known for their potent antioxidant qualities, they have antiviral, antihistaminic, anti-carcinogenic, and anti-inflammatory properties and are involved in immune function and maintaining the integrity of capillaries and connective tissue. Pine bark and grape seed oil are popular sources for flavonoid supplements. Eriksen (2004) believes that flavonoids can play an important role in preventing a chain of chemical reactions that can cause emotional or mechanical stress-induced muscle pain to become chronic.

Minerals

Magnesium: Because FM patients tend to have low levels of magnesium (Cox, Campbell, and Dowson 1991), magnesium is one of the most frequently recommended supplements for FM and CFS. Magnesium is a crucial contributor to the production of ATP—the body's energy currency—neurotransmitter function, and the action and repair of muscles. Magnesium deficiency is more likely to show itself in tests of red blood cell magnesium content than in serum levels. According to Podell (2003), pain and emotional distress cause the body to excrete magnesium. When magnesium is low, pain is increased. With increases in pain, more magnesium is lost, creating a vicious cycle. Magnesium's ability to raise energy levels is improved when combined with malic acid (Russell et al. 1995). It's important that magnesium be kept in balance with calcium.

Calcium: Although people primarily think of calcium in terms of its ability to build strong bones, calcium is also involved in protein and fat digestion, energy production, nerve transmission, neuromuscular activity, and the absorption of other nutrients, such as vitamin B_{12}. Together, calcium and magnesium regulate the contraction and relaxation of muscle tissue. Magaldi et al. (2000) believe a calcium-magnesium imbalance could be a major factor in the muscle pain of FM. Calcium citrate is a form that is often recommended, although if bone density is an issue, calcium hydroxyapatite seems to be the preferred form. Excessive intake of protein can lower the body's ability to absorb calcium, and the phosphorus in carbonated drinks can pull calcium from the bones, creating a risk for osteoporosis. Lund-Olesen and Lund-Olesen (1994) suggest that muscle pain in FM may be due to increased calcium in muscle tissue, but this hypothesis hasn't been tested yet.

Zinc: Zinc regulates the release of growth hormone, as well as protein synthesis, muscle contraction, healing, and mental alertness (Mindell and Mundis 1994). Zinc is also involved in immune and muscle function. By supporting the thymus gland, zinc affects the body's ability to fight illness. People with FM and CFS are often deficient in zinc; this deficiency is sometimes indicated by white spots on fingernails (Werbach 2000). Rogers (1990) believes zinc deficiencies may be more common in chemically sensitive individuals. Krotkiewski et al. (1982), investigating the role of zinc in muscle pain and fatigue, found supplementation helpful in healthy subjects for increasing strength and endurance. However, oversupplementation with zinc can decrease immune function and deplete copper.

Iron: Iron is integral to energy production and the transport of oxygen to cells. Iron deficiency can lead to decreased immune function. Iron deficiency—or a problem utilizing iron—can also be a cause of restless leg syndrome. Since both too-high and too-low iron levels can be problematic—and have similar symptoms—a lab test should be done to accurately determine iron levels and related factors. It's sometimes suggested that iron be taken with vitamin C to increase absorption (Sharma and Mathur 1995).

Trace Minerals

Molybdenum: Molybdenum deficiencies are rare; however, since molybdenum is important in the process of detoxification, a deficiency could be a causal factor in candida overgrowth and chemical sensitivities. For example, most Americans consume sulfites—a type of food preservative—on a regular basis. To metabolize sulfites, we need sulfite oxidase—which depends upon molybdenum (Pizzorno and Murray 2006). If we're deficient in molybdenum, we may become sensitive to sulfite-containing foods (Papaioannou and Pfeiffer 1984). Similarly, if we lack molybdenum, we may have difficulty breaking down byproducts of yeast and other toxins. Molybdenum is also involved in the breakdown of copper; excess copper is sometimes seen in people with FM or CFS.

Potassium: Potassium maintains both the body's fluid balance and its acid/base balance. It's also involved in metabolism, growth, and building muscle. Potassium must be kept in balance with other electrolytes—especially sodium—as well as with magnesium and calcium. No research is currently available on the effects of potassium supplementation in people with FM or CFS.

Selenium: Selenium is an important component of enzymes that have antioxidant properties and support the detoxification function of the liver. Other selenium-related enzymes regulate immune and thyroid function (NIH Office of Dietary Supplements 2004). Selenium intake from food depends on the level of selenium present in the soil in which foods are grown; supplementation is often needed. Reinhard et al. (1998) found lower levels of selenium in people with CFS compared to controls. According to Beck, Levander, and Handy (2003), selenium deficiencies make the body more vulnerable to nutritional, biochemical, and infectious stressors. Benton and Cook (1991) found that selenium supplementation had a beneficial effect on anxiety, depression, and fatigue in a nonpatient population. Pizzorno and Murray (2006) state that there is a greater need for selenium in elderly people and that combined with vitamin E, supplements lead to improvements in both fatigue and psychological variables.

Chromium: Chromium supports the regulation of blood sugar. Vitamin C and niacin improve the digestive tract's normally inefficient absorption of chromium. However, infection, stress (Anderson 1994), and consumption of sugar (Kozlovsky et al. 1986) all tend to deplete chromium. Anderson (1997) found that chromium had a normalizing effect on hypoglycemia—often a problem for people with FM and CFS, particularly those with adrenal fatigue. Chromium picolinate appears to be the preferred formulation.

Sodium (salt): Werbach (2000) suggests that for people with orthostatic hypotension (low blood pressure, particularly when standing up—commonly associated with adrenal fatigue), a moderate increase in salt intake from food may be helpful.

Digestive Aids

Digestive enzymes: Enzymes are proteins that enable and accelerate a variety of chemical reactions in the body. Enzymes such as pepsin, papain, protease, lipase, chymotrypsin, lactase, amylase, and pancreatin assist in digestion. Each enzyme specializes in a specific macronutrient (protein, fat, or carbohydrate). When enzymes aren't present in optimal quantities, supplementation with plant-based enzymes can help our bodies break food into nutrients. Production of some digestive enzymes tends to decrease with age, poor diet, and stress; some people may also have genetic tendencies to enzyme deficiency. No research is currently available on the effectiveness of enzyme supplementation in people with FM and CFS, but digestive problems are very common and anecdotal reports indicate that digestive enzymes can be helpful.

Probiotics: Probiotics are bacteria that normally live in the gut and play important roles in immunity and digestion. Probiotics help the immune system by competing with unwanted organisms for nutrition and oxygen, and altering the acidity of the gut. They also fight pathogens by producing metabolic end products—such as hydrogen peroxide—that inhibit or damage pathogens. If there are too few probiotics—or too many pathogens—probiotics can no longer carry out these functions, and an overgrowth of pathogens like bacteria, yeast, or parasites can occur. As discussed in chapter 2, this is known as dysbiosis and is common in people with FM and CFS as well as those with inflammatory bowel disease (Logan, Venket, and Irani 2003). Both stress and the antibiotics used to treat bacterial diseases can kill friendly bacteria, causing an imbalance. Dysbiosis can lead to malabsorption of nutrients, immune suppression, increased allergies, and the release of toxins into the bloodstream. Supplementation with probiotics can help restore the balance of intestinal flora. Probiotics can be taken either orally or, in cases where candida, E. coli, or other organisms have caused urinary tract infections or vaginal yeast infections, in the form of vaginal suppositories (Pizzorno and Murray 2006). Common categories of probiotics are *lactobacillus* and *bifidobacterium*; often, in the names of specific species, just the first letter of the category is used as a prefix (e.g., *L. sporogenes*).

One difficulty with probiotic supplements is that some probiotics aren't able to survive the digestive process, and/or they can't adhere to the walls of the intestines as they need to in order to be effective. Choosing a product that is enteric-coated can help with this. When choosing a supplement, it's important to choose one that has active probiotic strains. Supplement producers will often state a minimum number of active organisms present and may recommend an optimal storage temperature to retain potency.

Hydrochloric acid: The process of digestion is aided by naturally occurring acids in the digestive tract. Acid in the digestive tract signals the pancreas to release enzymes and the gall bladder to release bile. It also discourages overgrowth of bacteria and parasites and allows maximum utilization of calcium and other nutrients (Kelly 1997a). Many people mistakenly attribute digestive distress to excess acid when it's more likely that an acid deficiency is responsible. Sometimes, due to age, genetics, poor diet, or overuse of antacids or other pharmaceuticals, there isn't enough acid to properly digest foods, particularly proteins. In these cases, betaine hydrochloric acid or other forms of hydrochloric acid can help digestion. Kelly (1997a) states that thyroid disease and various skin conditions tend to correlate with low intestinal acid. Betaine also plays an important role in the synthesis of amino acids, B vitamins, and SAMe.

Amino Acids

The building blocks of protein, amino acids serve many functions in the body, including energy regulation, muscle repair, metabolism, digestion, and neurotransmitter control. Some amino acids, called *essential amino acids*, must be derived from food; *nonessential amino acids* can be synthesized by the body. Some of these, listed below, appear to have specific applications in FM and CFS. However, proper amounts of all of the amino acids are necessary for good health; tests are available to determine your amino acid profile.

Cysteine: Cysteine is a precursor to glutathione; glutathione is critical to cell metabolism and immune function. Droge and Holm (1997) suggest that supplementation with both cysteine and glutathione may be useful in immune dysfunction.

Glutathione: An antioxidant, glutathione is increasingly being recognized for its important role in many aspects of health. Bounous and Molson (1999) hypothesize that competition for glutathione precursors may be a causal factor in CFS. It's not clear whether supplementation is effective. So far, oral doses aren't effective, though a new form holds promise of effective oral absorption; glutathione can be given intravenously or intranasally, by prescription. SAMe and milk thistle supplements can increase glutathione levels.

Carnitine: Carnitine is needed for proper mitochondrial function. Kelly (1998) suggests that supplementation with carnitine may improve endurance. Plioplys and Plioplys (1997) found favorable effects with carnitine supplementation compared with a pharmaceutical used for treating fatigue in people with MS, among other conditions. In comparing two forms of carnitine in CFS patients, Vermeulen and Scholte (2004) found that acetylcarnitine was more effective for mental fatigue and propionylcarnitine was more effective for general fatigue.

Leucine, isoleucine, and valine: These three amino acids—known as *branched chain amino acids* (BCAA)—regulate protein synthesis and supply energy to the muscles. Lower concentrations of BCAAs and phenylalanine—another amino acid—have been found in people with FM (Maes et al. 2000). Maes and colleagues believe supplementation with these amino acids is justified, but no research as of yet attests to the results of such supplementation. Kelly (1997b) found that BCAA supplementation in athletes may have a sparing effect on muscle protein and glycogen, and that supplementation has a measurable effect on BCAA levels in plasma and BCAA uptake by muscles.

Tyrosine: One animal study indicates that tyrosine may be helpful in reducing fatigue and improving exercise tolerance, mood, thyroid function, and appetite (Avraham et al. 2001). Another study found tyrosine may improve cognitive functioning in fatigued people (Deijen et al. 1999).

Tryptophan and 5HTP: Tryptophan is involved in the production of serotonin—central to both pain and depression. Tryptophan is a precursor to the production of 5HTP, which is, in turn, involved in serotonin production (Birdsall 1998). 5HTP can cross the blood-brain barrier and has a number of other advantages in terms of the body's ability to utilize it. Simultaneous supplementation with magnesium and B_6 can help convert tryptophan to serotonin. Werbach (2000) cites ample evidence that tryptophan levels are low in people with FM and CFS, and Caruso et al. (1990) found beneficial effects from 5HTP in people with FM. Juhl (1998) states that repeated studies have shown tryptophan and 5HTP useful for depression, anxiety, pain, and sleep problems.

Glutamine: Glutamine is the preferred energy source for the cells lining the gastrointestinal tract. During times of stress, glutamine isn't synthesized as easily. Glutamine supplementation may benefit CFS patients (Kingsbury, Kay, and Hjelm 1998), and can be helpful in depression.

Gamma-aminobutyric acid (GABA): GABA is the most common neurotransmitter in the brain. Deficiency causes anxiety, irritability, depression, and sometimes insomnia. Anecdotally, supplementation with

GABA has a mild sedative effect and may relieve chronic pain in some people but not others. GABA is also thought to regulate levels of growth hormone produced by the pituitary. For supplementation to be effective, GABA would have to reach the brain; so far no research indicates whether it actually does. According to Jasmin et al. (2003), GABA may also play a role in alleviating pain by blocking the transmission of the brain's pain signals.

Dimethylglycine (DMG): DMG, a nonprotein amino acid, assists in the conversion of choline to glycine. It's also said to improve blood sugar regulation and has been used for many years by people eager to increase cellular oxygenation. However, as of yet no research supports these uses.

Hormones

Melatonin: A hormone secreted by the pineal gland during the night, melatonin regulates sleep-wake cycles. Melatonin also has antioxidant properties (Hardeland 2005), and plays a role in regulating the immune system (Brzezinski 1997). One recent study (Song et al. 2005) found melatonin effective in treating IBS when accompanied by sleep disorders— a combination often found in FM and CFS—though it had no impact on mood or the sleep problems themselves. Korszun et al. (1999) found that people with FM had higher levels of melatonin than controls; this was not the case for CFS. Based on their results, they believe melatonin supplementation in FM and CFS is inappropriate. This is a very controversial finding, counter to the experience of many health professionals who treat people with FM and CFS.

Dehydroepiandrosterone (DHEA) and dehydroepiandrosterone sulphate (DHEA-S): Produced primarily by the adrenal glands, DHEA regulates immunity, helps maintain the integrity of the immune system, and has antiviral qualities. DHEA is a precursor to sex hormones involved in memory, stress, anxiety, sleep, and depression. DHEA levels decline with age. DHEA levels are abnormal in certain characteristic ways in both CFS and depression (Scott, Salahuddin, et al. 1999). One study speculated that DHEA deficiency might be related to CFS symptoms (Kuratsune et al. 1998) and found that DHEA supplementation improved energy levels in CFS patients. Another study of DHEA levels in CFS patients found normal DHEA levels, but that less DHEA than expected was released by the adrenal glands when patients were given doses of adrenocorticotropin hormone—which normally causes the adrenal glands to secrete DHEA (De Becker et al. 1999). Scott, Svec, and Dinan (2000) had slightly different findings in response to the same challenge, with an altered ratio of DHEA and cortisol in the CFS group compared to the controls. So although these results are not well understood, it seems that there are differences in how DHEA operates in people with FM and CFS; it's not clear yet whether supplementation will help. Those with an adrenal component to their illness are more likely to respond to DHEA supplementation.

Other Types of Supplements

Essential fatty acids (EFAs): EFAs serve multiple functions in the body, including inflammation reduction, hormone production, mood regulation, immune function, and nerve function. Fish oil, flaxseed oil, hemp seeds, walnuts, black currant seed oil, and evening primrose oil are all good EFA sources. There are two types of EFAs: omega 3 and omega 6. The proper balance between them is important. Many people eat too many omega-6 fats and not enough omega-3 fats, creating an imbalance that makes them prone to a number of health problems, many of which are common in FM and CFS (Gray and Martinovic 1994). Randomized clinical trials showed significant improvement in CFS with EFA supplementation (Grey and Martinovic 1994). However, Warren, McKendrick, and Peet (1999) failed to replicate these results. One recent study also indicates that specific omega-3 fatty acids play a role in moods. Low levels of linolenic acid (LNA) were linked to being more impulsive, while low levels of eicosapentaenoic acid (EPA) and docosahexaenoic acid (DHA) were found in people who were more depressed (Conklin 2006). In a small study using EPA to treat people with CFS, Puri (2004) found that all of the participants reported overall improvement in CFS symptoms.

SAMe (S-adenosylmethionine): SAMe promotes cell growth and repair and has anti-inflammatory properties. It also assists in the synthesis of the neurotransmitters dopamine and serotonin and helps the body maintain glutathione levels—which in turn aids free radical elimination. Research has found SAMe comparable to antidepressants in relieving depression, with fewer side effects and faster action (Bressa 1994). It also aids in pain relief. Tavoni et al. (1987) found that SAMe reduced depression in FM patients, with a corresponding decrease in number of painful trigger points. However, in a short-term study, Volkmann et al. (1997) found no benefit to SAMe for pain or well-being when compared to a placebo. Jacobsen, Danneskiold-Samsoe, and Andersen (1991) found mixed results on the effectiveness of SAMe, with pain helped more than mood.

Phosphatidylserine (PS): Found in all cells of the body, with significant concentrations in the brain, PS is a fat-soluble substance that assists in cell repair and proper nerve signal transmission. PS naturally occurs in soy and egg yolks. PS has been found useful in cognition, memory, and mood (Pizzorno and Murray 2006). Most of the research on PS has been done with older people or those with dementias, but it's speculated that PS could be effective for the brain fog associated with FM and CFS. Monteleone et al. (1992) found that PS can help normalize the body's stress response, though this research wasn't done with FM or CFS patients. Anecdotally, PS seems to be helpful in FM and CFS.

Phosphatidylcholine (PC or lecithin): A fat-soluble substance quite similar to PS, phosphatidylcholine is a major constituent of cell membranes. PC enables the brain to produce neurotransmitters and is the body's main source of choline, an important nutrient. PC has been shown to help heal liver damage and protect the digestive tract from the adverse effects of aspirin and NSAIDs by maintaining the structural integrity of the intestinal wall (PC monograph 2002). Although claims have been made of cognition-enhancing properties, research does not support these claims (PC monograph 2002).

Glandular extracts: Derived from the glands of animals—usually cows or pigs—these extracts are believed to enhance the function of the same glands in humans. The glandular extracts most commonly used in FM and CFS are thyroid, adrenal, pancreas, and thymus. The theory is that ingesting glandular tissue will provide the body with the hormones and enzymes needed to support that gland in the human body. Some people have argued that after undergoing the digestion process the important constituents of the glandular products can't possibly be active; Gardner's work (1988) indicates that it is possible for the proteins to survive digestion. Because thyroid dysfunction is frequently found in people with FM and CFS—and because people with these illnesses can be hypersensitive to pharmaceuticals—a glandular extract of porcine thyroid gland is often used to normalize thyroid function. Armour Thyroid, the most common brand of this extract, is said to provide replacement of not only the T4 thyroid hormone, but also T3, the biologically active hormone. Some say this is unnecessary because the body can convert T4 into T3, but anecdotal evidence indicates that supplying it may be helpful as some people don't seem to be able to make the conversion. Whole adrenal and adrenal cortex extracts are said to be critical in addressing adrenal burnout, normalizing stress response, and regulating blood sugar. Thymus extract is used to improve immune function, and pancreas extract is used to assist digestion (Haas 2006). As you may imagine, it's crucial to use properly prepared products from healthy animals.

Creatine: Synthesized from three amino acids, creatine is often used by athletes to enhance their performance. Low levels of creatine have been found in people with FM (Park et al. 1998), and although there's no research as of yet on the effectiveness of creatine supplements in people with FM and CFS, research that shows an increase in ATP with supplementation suggests that supplements may be helpful in FM and CFS (Tarnopolsky, Roy, and MacDonald 1997). Schedel et al. (2000) found that creatine supplementation increases levels of growth hormone as much as vigorous exercise does, and Rae et al. (2003) found that creatine supplementation improves memory and cognitive processing speed.

Alpha lipoic acid (ALA): ALA plays a crucial role in the health of mitochondria, the energy centers of the body. When there's an excess of ALA, it acts as an antioxidant. A unique quality of ALA is that it is said to restore the antioxidant powers of other antioxidants, such as vitamins C and E. ALA also assists the B vitamins in creating energy from food. ALA supplementation improves control of blood sugar, diabetic neuropathy (Ziegler et al. 2004), and the central nervous system effects of heavy metal toxicity, and increases production of glutathione (Smith et al. 2004). Studies in rats indicate that when carnitine is combined with ALA, it has a rejuvenating effect (Ames 2003) and improves memory (Liu et al. 2002).

Ribose: Gebhart and Jorgenson (2004) have suggested that ribose, a carbohydrate used by the body in the production of ATP and RNA, can increase energy in people with FM and CFS. Their case report found supplementation led to improvement in sleep, mental alertness, joint pain, and bowel function for a patient with FM.

Medicinal mushrooms: Some mushroom varieties have immune-enhancing properties that work against viruses, bacteria, and fungi. This effect seems to be due, in part, to their *polysaccharide-protein complexes*, or *beta-glucans*. Polysaccharides are carbohydrates that increase macrophage function in the body. Some varieties of mushrooms are said also to increase oxygen uptake and assist in blood sugar regulation. Some of the mushrooms in use for these purposes are *Agaricus blazei*, reishi, maitake, *Cordyceps sinensis*, and shiitake. Many scientific studies attest to their effectiveness.

Chlorella pyrenoidosa: A single-cell green water plant, chlorella is rich in chlorophyll and may improve immune function and assist in detoxification. In one study of chlorella supplementation, patients with FM and ulcerative colitis reported reductions in pain and increases in quality of life (Merchant and Andre 2001).

CHAPTER 7

Herbal Therapy

People have used plants for healing since the beginning of time. Every society has had gifted people in tune with the properties of various plants; their wisdom has been passed down from generation to generation. In many cultures—and at most times in history—herbs have been at the center of healing practices; in many places this continues today. Thus, a rich tradition of herbal knowledge persists and is available to us.

One of the main characteristics of herbal therapy—also called phytotherapy, herbology, or botanical therapy—is that it treats the whole person. Although scientists have identified some of the specific compounds in herbs thought to be the active force behind healing, there is much that is not yet understood about the way plants heal. Because individual plants tend to contain a variety of compounds that work together to support health, traditional herbalists don't believe isolating specific compounds to be a helpful approach.

Medicinal plants can be used to treat problems with all fourteen elements of health. Since herbs are part of the practice of traditional Chinese medicine and ayurveda, it wouldn't make sense to take additional herbs if you're using these approaches. Herbs may also be used by an applied kinesiologist; tell him or her about any herbs you've been taking. Herbal care fits nicely with massage therapy and other forms of bodywork and energy work and can be a good support for psychotherapy, biofeedback, and nutritional approaches.

Quality and Purity

As with other nutritional supplements, quality is important—and varies tremendously from one product to the next. The guidelines in chapter 6 for finding the best quality nutritional supplements apply to herbs as well. Here are some additional things you should know that apply specifically to herbs.

An herbal product is only as good as the plant it is made from. One good option is *wild-crafted* plants—plants gathered in their natural habitats—which may have naturally ideal growing conditions, leading to heartier plants with more healing ability. Lately, though, cultivated plants are also being grown with the best of organic growing methods; these plants lead to good quality products—and using them prevents the depletion of scarce supplies of wild plants. However, all plants may be subject to the drift of pesticides or pollution. Also, most plants are at their best at certain times of the day and year; ideally, the plants in your herbal supplements will be gathered at those times. If plants aren't handled properly, they may be contaminated with other plants, molds, or insects. They may also lose important constituents and subtle energetic properties. Ethical suppliers have in-house labs that guarantee quality.

Potency

Herbal preparations guaranteed to have a set amount of an identified active component in them are referred to as *standardized*. Standardization is becoming more and more common and can be helpful—with standardization you know you're getting the intended dose of the herb. However, it can also be a problem. Because standardization sometimes isolates a single active ingredient from the plant's other synergistic components, it may render the herb less effective for whole-body healing. And because with most plants it's not yet known which components are crucial, key components may be lost in the standardization process. Also, the preparation of standardized extracts usually requires the use of chemical solvents, which can leave toxic residues in the finished product.

Although scientists who study herbs tend to believe that delivering a concentrated form of an herb's active constituent offers the best chance of successful treatment, many herbalists feel this approach renders herbs less effective. In some health care traditions—and for some health conditions—the potency of an extract is less important than retention of the *vital energy* of the plant. Vital energy refers to the life force present in all living things, a life force herbs can convey to strengthen a person's own subtle energy. Chapter 9, the chapter on homeopathy, will explain this in greater detail.

Interactions

Herbs can interact with other supplements and medications. As discussed in chapter 6, it's important to consult interaction databases to be sure that you aren't considering a dangerous combination. However, these databases are incomplete; until we have databases that are completely reliable, consulting a practicing herbalist with a wealth of experience is probably the best way of knowing the likely effects of a given combination.

Forms of Herbal Remedies

Different parts of the plants and different preparation methods produce remedies that have different healing properties. The following are some of the forms most commonly used:

Decoctions: Plant matter is simmered in water and then strained; the resulting liquid is consumed like a tea. This process is usually used with the roots, stems, or tough leaves. Decoctions and teas are the safest forms of herbs for self-care.

Teas or infusions: The leaves or flowers of a plant are steeped in hot water; the resulting liquid is strained and then drunk.

Extracts: Plant matter is treated with solvents—such as alcohol—to concentrate the effective portion of the plant. This is then prepared in a variety of ways, including tinctures, fluid extracts, and solid extracts. Because extracts are more concentrated, they hold more potential for harm.

Whole plant: The plant may also be used fresh or dried, without any extraction or concentration process. For example, fresh dandelion greens may be added to a salad as a springtime detoxifying tonic. Often plants are dried and then packed into capsules for efficient use. However, many herbalists believe that encapsulating herbs makes it difficult for our bodies to make the best use of them and may actually be dangerous.

Essential oils: Volatile oils that usually create the scent of a plant, these can be extracted by various methods to arrive at the concentrated "essence" of the plant. Essential oils are usually inhaled or applied to the skin rather than taken orally.

Balms: Ointments or salves made from herbs in an oily or creamy base, balms are for external application only.

Herbs and Their Actions

Because different plants grow in different places, herbal healing knowledge tends to differ from region to region—e.g., traditional Chinese medicine practitioners use different herbs than do Native American healers. Nowadays, we can benefit from the wisdom of people around the world, although some believe the herbs grown in one's own locale will be the most suitable ones. Despite regional differences, practitioners from most herbal traditions categorize the curative qualities of herbs in a similar way—according to the body processes the herbs support. The following is a selected listing of herbs with qualities helpful for FM and CFS. Because most herbs have several different ways of helping restore health, you will see some herbs listed more than once. In addition, many herbs work well in combination; some products will combine the ones that work best together.

Adaptogen

Adaptogen herbs have the unique ability to balance whatever is out of balance, particularly the body's responses to stress. Adaptogens tend to support the nervous and immune systems, particularly the adrenal glands. As you might imagine, this category of plants is very useful for FM and CFS where stress response is central to the problem. Examples: Siberian ginseng, American ginseng, ashwaganda, oat straw, rhodiola rosea, and licorice.

Sedative

Sedative herbs have a calming effect on the nervous system and can aid in sleep problems. For people with FM and CFS whose nervous systems seem to be stuck in the on position, these herbs can be very helpful indeed. Examples: passionflower, valerian root, chamomile, hops, skullcap, kava kava, and Saint-John's-wort.

Stimulant

Stimulant herbs increase energy and stimulate other aspects of functioning; this can be very useful for people who suffer from chronic fatigue. Examples: oat straw, ginger, ashwaganda, ginkgo biloba, licorice root, dandelion root, and Siberian ginseng.

Carminative

Carminative herbs help rid the body of excess intestinal gas—a main symptom of irritable bowel syndrome, often seen in conjunction with FM and CFS. Examples: peppermint, ginger, fennel, fenugreek, and chamomile.

Demulcent

Demulcent herbs soothe irritated mucous membranes; they are helpful for people who suffer from irritable bowel syndrome. Examples: burdock, aloe vera juice, marshmallow, slippery elm, colts-foot, and comfrey. (Some people are concerned about a class of toxic chemicals called *pyrrolizidine alkaloids* that have been found in colts-foot and comfrey; however, experienced herbalists continue to use them safely.)

Analgesic (Anodyne)

Analgesic herbs reduce pain; different herbs have different mechanisms of action and may be effective for different kinds of pain. Examples:

ginger, skullcap, turmeric, feverfew, cayenne, black cohosh, white willow bark, Saint-John's-wort, topical wintergreen oil, and topical cayenne.

Anti-Inflammatory

Although FM and CFS aren't primarily inflammatory processes, inflammation may play a role in the syndromes' secondary symptoms. Anti-inflammatory herbs can reduce pain and soothe the inflammation of irritated intestines. Examples: ginger, cat's claw (una de gato), licorice, poke root, pine bark, boswellia, and turmeric.

Immune Enhancing (Antiviral/Antibacterial)

Immune-enhancing herbs either directly strengthen the body's ability to fight off viruses and bacteria, or reduce the load on the immune system by killing organisms or inhibiting their growth. Examples: garlic, echinacea, goldenseal, burdock, pau d'arco, poke root, astragalus, ginger, grapefruit seed extract, schizandra berry, ashwaganda, gotu kola, chaparral, sangre de grado, cat's claw, olive leaf, aloe vera, and grape seed extract.

Cleansing/Detoxifying

Cleansing herbs help rid the body of excess toxins, either by helping to expel them from the body or by strengthening the body's ability to filter and detoxify them. Examples: red clover, sage, burdock, dandelion, milk thistle, poke root, turmeric, pine bark, grape seed extract, artichoke, Oregon grape, stillingia, and schizandra.

Fungicidal

Fungicides can help control overgrowths of yeasts and other fungi that sometimes occur in people with FM and CFS. Examples: oregano oil, pau d'arco, tea tree oil, and garlic.

Antidepressant

Saint-John's-wort is an herb that increases the availability of serotonin in the brain. For mild to moderate depression, Saint-John's-wort has been shown to be as effective as pharmaceutical antidepressants and is by far the most commonly used herb for depression.

How to Select Herbs

Because herbs are available over the counter, they can be used for self-care. Armed with some good resources, people can educate themselves about which herbs would be most applicable to their symptoms, in what form and what dose. A wealth of information is available about the safety and effectiveness of herbs, due in large part to the work of a German governmental group called Commission E, which undertook a massive study of the literature on 380 different herbs, and wrote thorough reports on their findings. These reports have also been published in English as *The Complete German Commission E Monographs: Therapeutic Guide to Herbal Medicines* (Blumenthal and Busse 1998). Because these monographs don't include some of the herbs most commonly used in the U.S., another very useful book is the *PDR for Herbal Medicines* (Medical Economics, Gruenwald, and PDR staff 2004), which is based on the Commission E monographs, but extends their reach. There are also searchable online databases that can help you learn what you need to know (see the Resources section at the end of the book).

Choosing a Practitioner

Experienced herbalists can guide you through the process of finding the most effective herbs for your health condition while avoiding possible harm. People knowledgeable about the use of herbs include naturopaths, chiropractors, holistic MDs, and traditional Chinese medicine (TCM) practitioners, as well as lay practitioners. Although a license guarantees a certain level of clinical competence in a practitioner, this doesn't necessarily hold true for their herbal practice as well. For example, most chiropractors don't have extensive knowledge of herbal therapy, although chiropractors are qualified to diagnose and treat many health conditions. The only governmentally approved credentials that reliably certify ompetence in herbal practice are the TCM herbal license—available only in some states—and the naturopathy degree, provided it's from one of the accredited schools of naturopathy. There are also voluntary credentials such as those offered by the American Herbalists Guild. However, even without a credential like a license or a degree, a person may still be well trained in herbal practice—they may have trained at an excellent school of herbalism or they may have served an apprenticeship with a master herbalist. Because of the depth and breadth of their understanding of herbs, these traditional herbalists are often actually a better choice. As with most forms of medicine, it's helpful to get a recommendation from a trusted person in your community. You can also contact the American Herbalists Guild, Bastyr University of Naturopathy, or Phytotherapy Research Labs for a referral in your area (see the Resources section).

CHAPTER 8

Applied Kinesiology, Chiropractic, and Related Techniques

Applied kinesiology (AK) is a system of diagnosis and health care based on using muscle tests to ask your body what's wrong and how best to restore health. Muscle tests are used not only to pinpoint the source of a problem, but also as an indicator of whether a treatment—such as a nutritional supplement, an acupressure technique, or a chiropractic adjustment—facilitates a particular aspect of a person's health. Once a treatment has been applied, a muscle test can be used to assess its effectiveness.

To conduct a muscle test, a doctor places one of your limbs in a particular position determined by a combination of anatomy, physiology, and neurology, and applies pressure to the limb while you resist. If the limb remains strong under this challenge, it's assumed that whatever function is being tested is neurologically facilitated. If the limb gives way under the pressure, it's assumed that something has switched off the nerves connected with that body part and the systems it's involved with. This is usually referred to as a muscle *testing weak*; this is a misnomer— testing weak doesn't have to do with how strong you are, but rather how well your body is functioning. Even the strongest of bodybuilders may test weak if something is malfunctioning, and even the weakest of people can have a strong muscle test. Sometimes the response to a muscle test is subtle; practitioners must practice a long time to develop skill in reliably determining outcome—much in the way physicians learn to listen to subtle breath sounds to determine if there's a problem with lung function. When a muscle test is properly carried out by a skilled practitioner, it will reliably achieve predictable, clear results.

A number of things can cause a muscle to test weak. A weak muscle test indicates that the nerves that control that muscle aren't doing their job properly. Nerve function can be affected by joint dysfunction causing improper stimulation of the nerve receptors in the spine, cranium, or limbs; nutrient deficiency; food sensitivities; excess toxicity; endocrine problems; environmental pollutants; negative emotions; organ dysfunction; disturbance in the subtle energies of the body; and constriction of the flow of cerebrospinal fluid.

Over years of experience applied kinesiologists have gained an understanding of associations between certain muscles and certain organs or glands. A muscle testing weak may indicate a dysfunction in the associated organ or gland, although there also may be many other factors influencing the muscle. For example, if the quadriceps muscle in your leg tests weak, it could indicate suboptimal functioning of the small intestine. However, a quadriceps muscle might also test weak due to a postural problem. A test alone isn't enough to pinpoint the cause of the weakness. Additional testing must be done, with other AK techniques as well as standard methods of diagnosis such as history taking; X-rays and other imaging studies; blood, urine, saliva, stool, and hair analyses; and thorough physical exams. AK testing, though, is often able to pick up subtle imbalances before they become the bigger problems that show up in standard medical tests.

Considerable research has been done on the accuracy of AK testing procedures and on the efficacy of AK treatment techniques. The Web site of the International College of Applied Kinesiology maintains a bibliography of those studies.

Because AK usually incorporates a number of other healing modalities, it can stand alone as a comprehensive treatment system and isn't often combined with other treatments, with the exception of massage and psychotherapy—and aromatherapy, flower essences, and homeopathy if your applied kinesiologist isn't using them. AK and associated techniques can have a direct beneficial effect on problems with all fourteen elements of health, although its effect on spiritual wellness is usually more indirect.

The Triad of Health

A simple concept called the *triad of health* represents AK's holistic conceptualization of health. The triad of health is a triangle with the base representing structural (musculoskeletal) aspects of health and the two other sides representing chemical and emotional/cognitive aspects. These three aspects of health are inextricably interwoven; dysfunction in one is likely to affect the other two. Most health problems affect all three, particularly if left untreated, as the body's attempts to compensate can cause further dysfunction.

Here is an example of how the triad of health might be used to understand the symptoms of a person with CFS:

■ Susan's Story

Susan was nineteen-years-old when she first noticed that she was feeling tired a lot of the time. She assumed her fatigue was from carrying a full load of college courses while working part-time as a receptionist in a beauty salon and spending late nights with her boyfriend. She lived in a college dorm. For spring break, she headed home for some pampering. Her mother cooked for her and did her laundry—all Susan had to do was sleep, eat, and hang out with her high school friends. By the end of the week, she felt a little better. However, as soon as she resumed her normal routine, she became so tired that she was concerned she wouldn't be able to keep her grades up to her usual high standards. During the summer semester, she began having severe migraines and painful menstrual cramps, and was frequently ill with flu-like symptoms.

A friend referred Susan to a chiropractor. In addition to taking a complete history and performing a thorough physical exam, the chiropractor used AK techniques to assess Susan— and determined that Susan's liver and adrenal glands weren't functioning well and that Susan was therefore somewhat toxic (the chemical side of the triangle). The chiropractor also determined that Susan's emotional stress was exacerbating these problems, as well as affecting her sleep (the emotional/cognitive side of the triangle).

The chiropractor used acupressure to strengthen Susan's liver functioning and suggested that she stop eating some of the less healthy foods that had become a regular part of her diet since moving to the dorm, and replace those foods with ones that supported health more actively. He also neutralized some of Susan's painful perfectionist self-judgmental thoughts and gave her supplements for adrenal support. In addition, because tests indicated a need for realignment assistance, he adjusted her neck (the musculoskeletal base of the triangle). These treatments helped Susan regain her normal level of energy and eliminated the headaches, menstrual cramps, and flu-like symptoms.

Treatment Techniques

Applied kinesiologists utilize a wide range of treatment techniques. These include:

Myofascial Release Technique

As we discussed in chapter 2, the fascia is a network of filmy connective tissue that surrounds the organs and muscles in our bodies. If a muscle has suffered trauma, sometimes the surrounding fascia will tighten up and restrict the range of motion of that part of the body as a defense against further injury. Over time, due to the effects of trauma, chronically poor posture, inflammation, or repetitive motions, the fascia can lose flexibility and cause discomfort or pain—which will, in turn, affect functioning in other parts of the body. Health care practitioners use hands-on stretching, massaging, and movement of the patient's body, so that the fascia can be restored to a healthier, more flexible state.

Craniosacral Therapy

The skull is composed of separate bony sections that meet along lines known as *sutures*. Skull bones aren't fixed; actually, they move in relation to each other. The movements of skull bones not only control the flow of our cerebrospinal fluid, but also affect the functioning of our cranial nerves.

There's a relationship between the bones of the cranium and the top of the spine and the bones of the sacrum and coccyx—or pelvic area—at the bottom of the spine, due to the fact that the *meninges*—membranes that protect your nervous system—are attached to both areas. Dysfunction in one of these areas often leads to dysfunction in the other, and if this secondary dysfunction is left uncorrected, either treatments won't be effective or effective treatments won't last. Dysfunction in the cranium and sacrum can be corrected with gentle manual manipulations that release restrictions and restore normal function.

Chiropractic Adjustment

Just as restrictions in the fascia can cause symptoms in both the immediate vicinity of the restriction and further afield, so can a restriction in the normal movement of the spine. Because all nerves except the cranial nerves pass through the spine, any misalignment of the spine can adversely affect the function of the nerves—which can, in turn, affect many aspects of health.

Chiropractic adjustments are manipulations applied to the bones of the spine—and other joints—to restore proper positioning and movement. Chiropractors use many different techniques to determine when an adjustment is needed, not just AK; most chiropractors don't use muscle testing at all. As of yet, there hasn't been much research on the use of chiropractic treatments in FM or CFS; however, a few smaller studies have found symptom improvement in FM patients who have had chiropractic treatment (e.g., Hains and Hains 2000). There's also considerable anecdotal evidence as to chiropractic's beneficial effects.

Meridian Therapy

Some systems of healing, like traditional Chinese medicine, include a highly developed understanding of how life energy—or chi—flows through the body and affects every aspect of our functioning. The pathways along which this energy travels are called *meridians*. In some spots these meridians are close to the surface of the body; these are sometimes referred to as *acupuncture points*. When the flow of chi is disrupted, these acupuncture points can be stimulated in a number of ways to restore normal chi flow. (These techniques will be described further in chapter

Applied Kinesiology, Chiropractic, and Related Techniques   **119**

10, the chapter on traditional Chinese medicine.) Applied kinesiologists often use *acupressure* techniques to stimulate these acupuncture points. Acupressure involves firmly rubbing the sites of acupuncture points. Applied kinesiologists also use the meridian system in their diagnostic and treatment procedures and may take advantage of specific muscle, nutrient, and spinal bone associations with the meridians—associations which offer additional ways of learning which body systems are involved in symptoms and which therapies may help.

Nutritional Supplementation

The AK muscle test can also serve as a way to determine which nutritional supplements are likely to be most effective for a specific person. Although a vitamin such as vitamin C may be useful for nearly everybody, the amount, the type, and even the best brand of vitamin C is likely to vary, both from one person to the next and for a given individual over time. Applied kinesiology offers both a way to know which supplement to take, and a way to determine when it's time to discontinue it. Without this direct feedback from the body, people may take supplements that aren't necessary—or may even actually harm the body.

Dietary Changes

As discussed in chapter 2, people with FM and CFS are prone to food sensitivities. Applied kinesiology offers a convenient way to accurately determine which foods may be causing problems, and which are the most suitable for a given individual. The most common method of AK food testing involves placing a small amount of a specific food—or a specially prepared food concentrate—on the tongue and then testing an associated muscle. The test can serve either as a basis for designing your optimal diet or as part of a process to desensitize you to specific foods.

How to Choose an Applied Kinesiologist

In order to qualify as an applied kinesiologist, hundreds of hours of coursework must be undertaken. The International College of Applied Kinesiology (ICAK) assures the quality of courses and provides credentialing services. Applied kinesiologists can be certified as proficient in AK or they can attain a higher credential called a *diplomate*. Many AK doctors opt not to pursue the diplomate; they may still have excellent skills in AK. The ICAK can provide referrals to qualified practitioners, who are usually chiropractors but may be nurses or other health care professionals as well. Applied kinesiology courses only admit licensed health care professionals.

Some people call themselves kinesiologists and practice a vastly simplified form of the muscle test, but they aren't properly trained to use the muscle test—or to interpret and act upon the results. These practitioners should be avoided.

CHAPTER 9

Homeopathy

Homeopathy is based on a fundamentally different way of conceptualizing health than the model most of us are used to. As a system of healing it's so different, in fact, that it tends to inspire skepticism in people who are only familiar with today's scientific, biomedical approach to health care. In a nutshell, you could say that modern mainstream medicine operates on the idea that every health problem has a specific, concrete cause, and if we negate this cause by working against it, we will get better. With homeopathy, symptoms are seen as signs of the body healing itself; the job of the homeopath is to support this healing, not work against it. In homeopathy there's no need to look for a single cause shared by all people with FM and CFS. In fact, with homeopathy, it's the uniqueness of each person that provides the basis for the right remedy.

Generally, homeopathic treatments shouldn't be used if you're taking medication—medication can conflict with the effects of remedies. This is true, too, for certain herbs and supplements. And because homeopathy is a comprehensive health care system, other treatment modalities may not be needed. However, homeopathy can combine well with massage, biofeedback, and psychotherapy. Homeopathy can be used to treat all fourteen elements of health.

The Law of Similars

Homeopaths support the body's healing through the use of specially prepared remedies made from natural substances that, if given to a healthy person, would cause the same symptoms the sick person is experiencing.

These remedies, then, assist the body in doing what it has already begun, rather than try to make it stop what it's doing. This is referred to as the law of similars, or as "like cures like."

Central to the formulation of these remedies is a process called a *proving*. In a proving, a medicinal substance is ingested by one or more healthy volunteers and careful observations are made about what symptoms are induced by the substance. If the proving shows that a certain substance induces a headache, for instance, then that substance may be useful for a person who has a headache. But many homeopathic remedies induce headaches in provers. A remedy is more likely to be helpful to a patient with a headache if the other symptoms observed in the proving also closely match those of the patient. For example, if a patient's headache feels like a tight band around the head, was brought on by an emotional upset, and is accompanied by fatigue, poor sleep, a lack of thirst, dizziness, performance anxiety, and a fear of being injured, he or she would be most likely to benefit from a homeopathic remedy that caused all of these symptoms in the provers as well.

Since the founding of homeopathy two hundred years ago, so many provings have been carried out that just about any set of symptoms can be matched to a substance observed to elicit those symptoms. New provings are still being carried out today.

Treating the Whole Person

You may notice that of the symptoms listed above, some are physical in nature and some are emotional, cognitive, or spiritual. An important aspect of homeopathic care is that the right remedy addresses every aspect of a person's functioning. The target of treatment is the whole person, not just their symptoms. It has been said that the goal of homeopathy is the complete restoration of good health, so that the person isn't limited in any way, physically, emotionally, spiritually, or cognitively.

Homeopaths look for a remedy with characteristics that match your symptom totality, with the sole goal of finding the most effective remedy. In a way, the homeopath is a matchmaker. His or her job is to find the remedy that most closely matches the symptom picture of the patient. Two main tools are used to do this: taking the case and materia medica.

Taking the Case

A homeopath will spend a long time talking to you about your symptoms, your personality, your preferences, your genetic background, your thoughts, and your emotions. Careful observation will also be a part of the interview. This first visit is called *taking the case*; it provides the homeopath with a rich source of detailed information about you. The goal is for the homeopath to know you as well as possible, so that he or she can find the remedy that best matches your constitution. You can expect questions about your worldview; the content of your dreams; the times of day when you feel best or worst; your worries; the foods you crave or avoid; your preferred types of weather and terrain; whether you feel better standing, sitting, or lying down; the color and texture of various bodily secretions; the sound of your cough; etc. These are the kinds of things that provers of remedies reported on; your responses will assist the homeopath in the matchmaking process.

Materia Medica and Repertories

The results of provings are recorded in *materia medica*—listed by remedy—and *repertories*—listed by symptom. These reference tools list every detail of the shared experiences of the many provers who ingested a remedy. There are several different materia medica and repertories; most likely your homeopath will consult more than one of them. These days, many homeopaths use computer programs to search these reference tools. For instance, if a patient presents with neck pain, a homeopath can search either the indexes of the reference books or the reference databases on their computer for neck pain, thus beginning the process of finding the right remedy for that patient.

Classical vs. Symptomatic Homeopathy

The approach we've discussed—where the whole person is treated with a single remedy—is called *classical homeopathy*. Sometimes, another form of homeopathy is used that addresses single symptoms, or clusters of symptoms—such as seasonal allergies—using some of the same principles as classical homeopathy, but applying them less broadly. This is known as *symptomatic homeopathy*; although symptomatic homeopathy may lead to symptom relief, it doesn't achieve the kind of total restoration of health that classical homeopathy aims for. When using homeopathy to treat symptoms, sometimes combination remedies will be used in the hope that at least one of the constituents of the remedy will be the right one.

The Remedies

The preparation method of homeopathic remedies is another aspect of this healing art that stretches the credulity of many people. Homeopathic remedies are extremely diluted forms of natural substances. In fact, they are so diluted that in some cases not a single molecule of the original substance remains. Remedies, usually given Latin names, are prepared according to processes laid out in a manual called the *Homeopathic Pharmacopoeia of the United States*, recognized by the U.S. Food and Drug Administration.

A substance, let's say a plant, is made into a tincture by applying a solvent that extracts the active material from the plant; this tincture is then diluted by placing one drop of it in ninety-nine drops of distilled water. The mixture is then shaken vigorously—a process called *succussion*, which is said to activate the remedy. The potency of the resulting formula is called 1C. Next, one drop of this 1C dilution is added to ninety-nine drops of water and then succussed again, resulting in a dosage referred to as 2C. The more times the remedy is diluted in this manner, the more potent it becomes. After a few successive dilutions, the amount of the original active substance is so low as to be undetectable. However, homeopaths argue that these liquids retain the imprint or energy signature of the original material in a form that can be transferred to the body of the person who consumes it.

Remedies are either taken as drops of this liquid, or, more commonly, as small tablets or pellets saturated with the remedy—which are to be dissolved on or under the tongue. You might take a single dose or a daily dose of a homeopathic remedy, and then return to the homeopath a few weeks later to assess its effect. It may take several tries to find the best remedy for you. After a remedy has been effective, another one may be needed to treat a newly emerging symptom picture; it's rather like peeling away the layers of an onion.

Research

Two large *meta-analyses*—studies that examine the results of a number of other studies, to get an overview of the literature—have been published that support the efficacy of homeopathic remedies (Kleijnen, Knipschild, and ter Riet 1991; Linde et al. 1997). Another meta-analysis (Shang et al. 2005) concluded that the effects of homeopathy were due to placebo effect. All of these meta-analysis articles were published in top medical journals, and all of them inspired heated debates in the scientific literature. The two-hundred-year history of homeopathy is rich in anecdotal evidence of effectiveness.

Do-It-Yourself Homeopathy?

If you have the proper resources—and the ability and willingness to study—it's possible to treat yourself or a loved one with a homeopathic remedy. Most remedies can be purchased over the counter; some people invest in a kit that contains commonly used remedies. Self-treatment with homeopathy tends to be more focused on treating symptoms than on treating the whole person. Many reference materials are available to assist in your search. Although none of them are specific to FM and CFS, all include coverage of the symptoms of FM and CFS. Usually, taking the wrong remedy leads to no adverse effects. In some areas, peer study groups assist each other in determining correct remedies.

However, you're more likely to find the best remedy for your total health by working with a trained homeopath. Homeopaths may be licensed in one of the health care professions; it's a good idea to seek one who does have a license—they'll be able to recognize serious illnesses that need immediate medical intervention. Look for one who is a certified classical homeopath (CCH) or has one of the following credentials: a diplomate in Homeotherapeutics (D.Ht.—for physicians and osteopaths) or a diplomate of the Homeopathic Academy of Naturopathic Physicians (DHANP—for naturopaths).

CHAPTER 10

Traditional Chinese Medicine

Central to the understanding of traditional Chinese medicine (TCM) is the concept of chi—or life energy—that flows through the body along specific pathways called channels or meridians. Chi (also spelled qi) is often spoken of as if it were a tangible substance that can be seen and measured. This isn't actually the case, but does provide a useful way of talking about how it affects health. We are born with chi from our parents; when chi is depleted, we can restore it through the use of some of the treatments referred to below.

Traditional Chinese medicine is an ancient art and science that predates the invention of microscopes and modern imaging techniques by thousands of years, thus its methods of diagnosis necessarily entail aspects of functioning that can be seen and experienced from outside of the body. In TCM, a person's state of health is determined through pulse rhythms, body shape, skin tone, tongue condition, eye brightness, and careful analysis of the person's medical history and current symptoms.

TCM is a comprehensive health care system; no other healing modalities are usually needed along with it, although psychotherapy can complement it well. TCM is an approach that can be used to address all fourteen elements of health.

How Does It Work?

Even though the underlying principles of TCM are very different from those of Western medicine, many people have attempted to explain the results seen with TCM through the explanatory models of Western medicine. It has been hypothesized that TCM techniques alter levels of hormones and neurotransmitters, stimulate the constriction and dilation of blood vessels, and enhance immune system function by increasing the activity level of its components. It has also been hypothesized that acupuncture and other TCM techniques create a sensation that competes with pain, so that any pain is experienced as less severe.

TCM practitioners generally work within a rich conceptual framework based on Taoist philosophy, and don't attempt to explain what they do in Western medical concepts. TCM diagnosis involves describing—to our Western ears in a somewhat picturesque way—overall health status (called *zheng*) and any imbalances or disharmonies that exist in a person's body, mind, and spirit. The following concepts are used:

Yin and Yang

In TCM, the terms *yin* and *yang* are used to denote the opposing and complementary qualities shared by all things. Although opposites, they can't exist without each other, and each has a little bit of the other. For example, yin is associated with dark while yang is associated with light; yin is more feminine and yang is more masculine; yin is passive and yang is active; yin is inward and yang is outward; and so on. However, all of these terms are expressed in relation to each other, so warm water is yang relative to cold water, but yin relative to boiling water. With yin and yang, balance is key—treatments aim to restore lost balance.

Fundamental Substances

Fundamental substances include chi, blood, *jing* (a nutritive substance that supports development and change in the body), *shen* (spirit or vitality), and fluids such as sweat, saliva, and urine. The source of these fundamental substances is twofold: we are born with some and some come from food and other sources of nourishment. These fundamental substances may at times be insufficient, stagnant, blocked, or excessive, leading to health problems.

Organs

Many of the organs of TCM have the same names as the ones used in the West, but are thought to have somewhat different or more complex functions, including storing and directing the fundamental substances. Organ function can be impaired by a number of factors. These impairments are often described in terms of imbalances of yin and yang. Emotions, if too extreme, are thought to have predictable effects on the organs of the body. For example, excessive anger can cause liver chi to stagnate.

Environmental Factors

In addition to lifestyle factors and emotions, environmental factors are seen as a main cause of imbalance. These factors are spoken of in meteorological terms—e.g., wind, heat, cold, and damp—but these terms are used in a much more broad and complex way than we typically use them. These environmental factors are manifestations of chi from outside the body and may interfere with the body's own chi.

Treatment Methods

The goal of TCM treatments is usually to restore the proper flow of chi and other fundamental substances. This is accomplished through a variety of methods:

Acupuncture

Also called needling, acupuncture is the insertion of very thin needles at those points on the body where the meridians come close to the surface. These sterile needles rarely cause pain or bleeding, although sometimes they are accompanied by sensations such as tingling, stinging, or a dull ache that only lasts a moment. Sometimes, to increase stimulation, needles are manipulated after insertion by rolling them between the fingers, flicking them, or withdrawing them slightly. Some acupuncturists also apply mild electric currents to the needles to accomplish the same objective.

Acupressure

With acupressure, rather than inserting needles at acupuncture points, these points are instead manipulated by deep, focused massage with a thumb, finger, or a small instrument with a ball on the end.

Moxibustion

Moxibustion is the burning of an herb called mugwort (*ai ye* in Chinese) close to the acupuncture points on the skin. The heat generated by the smoldering herb stimulates the flow of chi. Moxibustion complements the use of acupuncture; usually the two are used together.

Tuina

Tuina is a method of bodywork unique to TCM. Its goal is the restoration of the normal flow of chi, rather than directly affecting tight or sore muscles and connective tissues as in Western massage therapy. It can be a fairly vigorous form of massage, involving firm pressure applied by elbows and thumbs as well as fingers and hands, and may include the application of poultices or salves as well.

Cupping

In *cupping*, a vacuum is created in a small cup or closed tube made of wood, glass, or bamboo; this cup is then placed on the surface of the body. The suction created by the vacuum draws blood to the surface, stimulating the body to heal.

Tai Chi and Qi Gong

By moving the body in specific ways, the flow of chi can be optimized. The slow, graceful movements of tai chi and qi gong follow forms established thousands of years ago; these practices allow people to cultivate and control their own chi to restore and maintain good health.

Herbs

The TCM herbalist can choose from thousands of single herbs and hundreds of ancient formulas for combination remedies. Traditionally, Chinese herbs are prescribed to address a specific state of disharmony; this prescription may change regularly as a patient's body changes.

Diet

Foods are believed to have unique proportions of yin and yang. Yin foods are sweet, cool, wet, and grow above the ground, while yang foods are salty, warm, dry, and grow under the ground. Some foods have a balance of yin and yang, while others are more extreme. Cooking methods can also affect the qualities of food. For good health, yin and yang must be kept in balance. If a person's health problem is caused by—or made worse by—too much of one or the other, choosing foods according to their yin or yang dominance can help to restore balance. This will result in dietary recommendations that are very different than the ones that most of us are used to, involving fats, calories, sugar, etc.

TCM and FM and CFS

Because TCM works with the overall constitution of an individual rather than with a disease entity, individuals with CFS and FM may have different descriptive diagnoses. Generally, though, FM and CFS are seen as due to deficiencies of the organs—particularly the kidneys, spleen, and liver—and to a deficiency of chi. For example, a person with FM or CFS might be described by a TCM practitioner as having "liver yin deficiency," or a "damp cold invading the spleen."

From the point of view of TCM, FM is due in part to a blockage of chi that affects the muscles. This is referred to as muscle *bi*. This may be due to environmental factors—e.g., wind, cold, and damp—that the body is unable to fight against due to a vulnerability created by genetics, diet, stress, overwork, lack of proper exercise, or other factors that interfere with the body's ability to maintain sufficient defenses.

A recent study (Singh et al. 2006) found that TCM helped reduce pain and depression in people with FM. A number of other studies show moderate support for the effectiveness of TCM for FM and CFS (e.g., Deluze et al. 1992; Berman et al. 1999). The National Institutes of Health has declared that acupuncture may be "useful as an adjunct treatment or an acceptable alternative or be included in a comprehensive management program for a variety of illnesses," including FM and myofascial pain (NIH 1998, 1522). A recent study conducted by Martin et al. (2006) showed that acupuncture helped people with FM, particularly in reducing fatigue and anxiety.

How to Choose a Practitioner

Schools of TCM are accredited by the Accreditation Commission for Acupuncture and Oriental Medicine, and generally involve several years of study—including supervised clinical practice—and lead to a master's degree. However, in some states physicians or chiropractors are permitted to practice acupuncture with substantially less training than this, and may use TCM techniques without grounding them in the philosophy of TCM. Most states offer a license specifically for the practice of TCM, although in some states the practitioner must also be licensed as a medical doctor. A few states also license practitioners of Chinese herbology. The NCCAOM (National Certification Commission for Acupuncture and Oriental Medicine) provides credentialing for practitioners of acupuncture, herbology, and oriental bodywork. Some states use these credentials as a basis for granting licenses, while other states have more challenging criteria for licensure. To locate a practitioner, first find out if your state has a licensing board for acupuncture; if so, this will be a good source of referrals to well-trained professionals. If not, you may want to visit the Web site of the NCCAOM for names of practitioners credentialed under their criteria.

Chapter 11

Therapeutic Massage

Many people think of massage as pampering, as a spa treatment intended simply to help a person relax and feel good. But massage is also a healing art and can have a significant impact on a variety of health problems, including FM and CFS. Massage therapy involves the manipulation of muscle and other soft tissue through the use of various kinds of touch. Specialized massage treatments may be directed toward the fascia, the chi (life energy), the cranial and sacral bones, the lymphatic system, or some other specific body part or system; more commonly, the whole body is treated.

Massage has a therapeutic effect on all fourteen elements of health and combines well with nearly any other healing technique, unless that technique already includes massage.

Types of Massage

There are many different styles of massage; these include:

Swedish massage: A popular massage technique that involves firm but gentle strokes that aim to relax muscles, increase flexibility, and improve circulation.

Shiatsu: Deep massage of the acupuncture points for healing.

Deep tissue massage: The use of firm, kneading strokes to reach deep levels of muscle and connective tissue. Deep tissue massage is often used to restore normal structure and function following an injury, and is believed, too, to release emotions held in the body from past events, including trauma.

Sports massage: Massage aimed to improve athletic performance, by keeping the body flexible and healing any injuries; sports massage may also include stretching techniques.

Lymphatic massage: Focused on the lymph nodes, lymphatic massage can restore the free flow of the lymphatic fluid, a crucial immune system component.

Reiki and related techniques: Sometimes referred to as the laying on of hands, reiki works with the energy field of the body. In energy work, the hands of the healer may just be held over the skin of the patient; sometimes light touch is involved.

Aromatherapy massage: Massage incorporating the use of scented oils selected according to their healing properties.

Reflexology: Massage of points on the soles of the feet that correspond to other parts of the body and stimulate healing in those areas.

Stone massage: A soothing massage that uses smooth stones—either cool or warm—that are placed on the back as a person lies face down.

Watsu: A popular new kind of massage that gently releases stress as a person floats in a warm pool.

The Power of Touch

Human beings thrive on touch. Infants that aren't touched will die. The touch of a massage therapist can help fulfill this basic human need. Field and colleagues (1997) found that for people who had experienced sexual or physical abuse, massage decreased aversion to touch. People who tend to focus their awareness on thoughts and feelings rather than physical sensations report that massage can get them back in touch with their bodies. This can be very important for people with FM and CFS.

Stress Reduction

Massage therapy has a proven track record of normalizing the stress response, which in turn allows the body to heal. Cortisol, one of the stress hormones, suppresses immune function; when cortisol levels are reduced, immune function improves (as measured by an increased number of natural killer cells, a critical component of immune functioning). Massage therapy has been shown to reduce cortisol levels. A study by Field et al. (2005) showed massage therapy led to clear changes in neurotransmitter action, toward a more relaxed state; research by Diego et al. (2004) found that massage brought about changes in brain waves and mood consistent with a relaxation response.

Pain Management

Several studies (e.g., Gordon, Emiliozzi, and Zartarian 2006) have found significant pain reduction, decreased depression, and improved quality of life for FM patients upon receiving massage therapy treatments. When pain levels are reduced, sleep improves—which enables the body's natural mechanisms of restoration and repair to function. *Substance P* is a neurotransmitter central to the experience of pain; levels of substance P are often high in people with FM. Field et al. (2002) found that massage decreased levels of substance P in people with FM.

Sleep and Fatigue

Field et al. (2002) reported that people with FM who received massage therapy had increased hours of sleep and less movement during sleep— as well as less pain, depression, and anxiety. Similar results have been mentioned in other studies of massage in people with FM and CFS.

Cognitive Function and Brain Fog

Field and colleagues (1996) used electroencephalogram (EEG) instruments to measure changes in brain waves after massage treatment and found that, compared to spending the same period of time just relaxing, massage brought about changes in brain function consistent with a more relaxed, more alert mental state. They also found a greater ability to perform mathematical tasks quickly and correctly and less depression and anxiety. Similarly, after receiving massage treatments, people with FM and CFS often report relief from brain fog.

Improved Blood and Lymph Circulation

The lymphatic system helps to clear toxins from the body and transports some of the components of the immune system. Sometimes, however, lymphatic fluid stagnates and doesn't do its job properly. Specialized massage techniques aim to normalize the functioning of the lymphatic system. According to Cassar (1999), massage can relieve symptoms that arise from toxins in the system—such as fatigue, body pain, constipation, and headaches—and can normalize immune function and cell oxygenation.

Finding a Massage Therapist

Most states regulate the practice of massage therapy, licensing only people who have met certain educational and ethical requirements. The exam offered by the National Certification Board for Therapeutic Massage and Bodywork is used in many states to establish competence. A recommendation from somebody you trust can also be very helpful. People can feel vulnerable during massage; a personal recommendation can increase your feelings of comfort and safety as you begin treatment. Personal recommendations can also help you find a massage therapist with a level of interaction that matches what you're looking for—some massage therapists are chatty, some maintain a complete silence, and some play relaxing music. It's important that the massage therapist you choose have some understanding of your illness; if you aren't sure they do, ask them. You can also ask them about their training and the kinds of massage techniques they use.

When you arrive for your first session, the massage therapist should talk to you about your health history and your current symptoms. This will help him or her develop a treatment plan that fits your situation. Next, he or she will probably step out of the room while you undress and get on the massage table. If you're uncomfortable with nudity, you can probably leave some clothes on. The massage therapist will drape a sheet, blanket, or towel over the parts of your body that aren't being worked on, and may provide pillows to help position your body more comfortably. Once the massage begins, you can give the massage therapist feedback about which techniques you like and don't like. Massage therapists often let intuition guide their work with different people and different parts of the body, but should also be attentive and responsive to their clients' needs and concerns.

It's important to know that some pain is associated with deep tissue massage techniques; without it, you may not be able to derive the full benefits of these approaches. However, because people with FM and CFS are sometimes hypersensitive to pain, a lighter touch may be needed. Also, massage oil or lotion may or may not be used. If you're sensitive to scents—or if you tend to get skin rashes—discuss this with the massage therapist before the massage begins. Even if a massage therapist doesn't use scented oil on you, the therapist's office may still be strongly scented from previous clients.

CHAPTER 12

Psychotherapy

You may have been told that your illness is "all in your head"—that if you decided to, you could just "snap out of it." This obviously isn't true, but in these misguided statements there is a kernel of truth that holds an important key to recovery. FM and CFS are due largely to a stress response that has gotten out of hand and begun to affect nearly every system of the body. Physical health is so intimately tied to emotional health and spirituality that when we make a change in any of these three areas, we typically also see changes in the other two. The bad news is that a difficulty in one of these areas can end up affecting all of them—and becoming a much bigger problem than it was at first. The good news is that when something goes wrong you have three different ways to intervene.

Psychotherapy is the primary way to work on the emotional part of the equation (although some people do quite well with self-reflection and other methods). Seeking psychotherapy doesn't mean you're crazy and it doesn't mean your illness isn't real. It just means that you're committed to using all the resources available to you to overcome your health problems.

Psychotherapy has a direct beneficial effect on emotional response, sleep and restoration, and—to some degree—spiritual wellness. Due to the interconnections between body and mind, it also has an indirect effect on all of the other elements of health. Psychotherapy combines well with other healing modalities, and generally should be just a single part of a health care plan including other methods. It can be particularly useful in handling emotions that arise during the course of bodywork. Some people feel that psychotherapy isn't necessary if you're using homeopathy, traditional Chinese medicine, or ayurveda since these modalities treat mental health concerns. However, many people who combine psychotherapy with these modalities find it useful. It wouldn't be a good idea to use more than one form of psychotherapy at a time, although being in group and individual psychotherapy can be a good combination.

Theoretical Models of Psychotherapy

Much in the way that all ice cream is cold, sweet, and creamy, but vanilla ice cream is different from pistachio, psychotherapy comes in different flavors. All forms of psychotherapy have the same aim and general method: use of confidential conversations between a trained professional and a help-seeker to bring about positive changes in one or more areas of the help-seeker's life. But there are a number of different ways to bring this about. Psychotherapy can occur in a group format, a couple or family format, or one-on-one. Also, different theoretical models underlie the practice of psychotherapy. The main models include cognitive therapy, insight-oriented therapy, behavior therapy, and hypnotherapy.

Cognitive Therapy

This flavor or model of therapy is based on the idea that behind every emotion is a causative thought. For instance, when you think that you may fail a test, fear is likely to result. If you also say to yourself—our thoughts often take the form of internal dialogue—"my parents will kill me if I fail this test," then your fear will probably be quite strong. If you don't know that you're having these thoughts, you may feel the fear is impossible to overcome. By becoming aware of these thoughts, you can choose to think different ones, such as "I may or may not fail this test. I've studied hard and done well on tests in the past. Even if I were to fail, my parents love me, and although they may temporarily be angry with me, they'll get over it." With this second set of thoughts, fear is now much less likely to be a dominant emotion. And less fear means the body doesn't have to be alert for a crisis; as a result, you'll probably think more clearly and perform better on the test. This type of change can be a big help in FM and CFS—if your body doesn't have to be on alert status, your health care is more likely to be effective.

Cognitive therapy aims to help you identify troublesome thoughts that lead to painful emotions and transform them into different

142

thoughts—or self-talk that is more accurate, less extreme, and more optimistic. A cognitive therapist will talk to you about what's on your mind while listening for the thoughts that underlie your emotions. When these thoughts have been identified, you'll work with the therapist to formulate and practice healthier thoughts—both in the session and between sessions—until you can do it on your own. Cognitive therapy combined with behavior therapy called cognitive behavioral therapy (CBT) has been shown to be a very effective treatment for FM and CFS (Goldenberg, Burckhardt, and Crofford 2004).

Insight-Oriented Therapy

Sometimes, the thoughts and feelings we habitually experience come from things that happened to us in the past. For example, if you grew up with parents who were quick to anger, you might be more likely to think, "my parents will kill me if I fail the test"—thus making you more prone to fear. If instead you had happy-go-lucky parents who never set limits on your behavior, you might be more likely to have a thought like, "I don't feel like taking this test today"—and your resulting emotion might be anger at having to be indoors taking a test on a beautiful day. Sometimes it's easier to change thoughts and emotions when we know their source. This is what insight-oriented therapy is all about. In insight-oriented therapy, you work with a psychotherapist trained to recognize patterns in your thoughts and feelings, who will help you trace them back to their origins in the past, empowering you to choose different responses.

Behavior Therapy

There are times when, instead of working to understand why you do something, it's helpful to simply find a way to stop doing it. For example, the test-anxious person mentioned above could train his or her body to relax, reducing or eliminating the fear response altogether. Similarly, although it may be helpful to understand why a person bites his or her nails, it may be more expedient simply to train the person to stop doing so by putting a foul-tasting substance on the nails that will make it unpleasant to bite them and eventually eliminate the behavior altogether. This is behavior therapy. In behavior therapy, the help-seeker and psychotherapist work together to identify problem behaviors and challenges that make these behaviors hard to stop. They then address these challenges to make the problem behaviors easier to change. For example, if a person with FM or CFS finds it impossible to stop eating unhealthy foods, behavior therapy can work to create a system of rewards and punishments so that eating healthier food is more rewarding and more likely to occur. Behavior therapy can also help you acquire specific skills—such as decision making, assertiveness, self-control, relaxation, and self-care—which may be crucial for your recovery.

Hypnotherapy

Hypnotherapy is a tool that can be used in nearly any model of psychotherapy. Hypnotherapy can assist you to identify thoughts and feelings, discover their roots, get in touch with preferences and dreams for the future, and change behaviors. Hypnotherapy can also be helpful in modifying physical symptoms—such as those associated with IBS. With hypnotherapy, a psychotherapist will help you bring a highly focused state of attention to the matter at hand, thus optimizing the use of your internal resources.

Common Issues for People with FM and CFS

Although there are emotional/cognitive patterns unique to each individual, certain patterns tend to be associated with FM and CFS. Here is a brief summary of common patterns and what psychotherapy can do to help:

Issues That Predate FM or CFS

People with FM and CFS may have a tendency toward perfectionism and overemphasize work and achievement over relaxation and pleasure. Although this approach to life has its rewards, it also has significant drawbacks, including high levels of stress; psychotherapy can help people move toward a more balanced approach.

Another experience commonly shared by people who have FM and CFS is childhood physical, emotional, or sexual abuse. This has a number of important consequences in terms of physical, emotional, and spiritual health. A history of abuse may cause life to seem frightening, out of control, or meaningless. You might also feel that your body and other aspects of who you are somehow aren't good enough. Through psychotherapy, a sense of safety can be restored and self-esteem improved; you can learn to find meaning and purpose in new ways.

If you have trouble identifying or really feeling your feelings—common among people with FM and CFS—you're cut off from the information you need to make good decisions in many areas of your life, such as relationships, food choices, career, etc. Psychotherapists are trained to help get you back in touch with your emotions and the way your body feels—which can give you the information you need to shape a life for yourself that's more to your liking. Through psychotherapy you can also gain skill in regulating your emotions so they feel less overwhelming.

If you use food to manage emotions, it can be very difficult to choose the right foods for best health. It's hard to just let yourself feel painful emotions; some people keep themselves so busy that they never have to feel them and some people develop addictions in an effort to manage them. When these obstacles to good self-care are removed, you're more able to achieve optimal health. Psychotherapy can help you find better ways to manage emotions.

Issues That Arise as a Result of FM or CFS

FM and CFS usually cause enormous change in people's lives; with change comes a number of psychological effects, including depression and anxiety. It's important to acquire adaptive coping mechanisms—there's a lot to cope with in FM and CFS. In addition to helping with depression and anxiety, psychotherapy can help with the following issues:

Relationships

It can be hard to maintain strong relationships when your ability to do what you used to do is compromised. In the quest for control over aspects of life that have suddenly become uncontrollable, maladaptive behavior may arise, either in relationships or in your own daily routines. Social support is crucial for your recovery, but it's not always easy to get. You may not have a partner or close family members. If you do have a partner, he or she may have to deal with his or her own issues about being called upon to take care of you, your possible lack of interest in sex, and the changing balance of power in the relationship. Children may feel afraid or neglected, leading to feelings of guilt on your part—even though you're doing the very best you can, given how ill you are. Finances can also become a major concern if you can't work due to your illness. You and your family might need to set new goals. Couples or family therapy can be helpful in improving relationships around the changes brought about by your illness.

For some people, an inability to work and achieve, to enjoy certain leisure time activities, or to serve loved ones in accustomed ways brings up identity issues, causing you to lose track of who you really are. When you've lost a significant part of the basis of your identity, it's only too easy to latch onto the role of FM or CFS patient as a new identity—not a good indicator for a fast recovery. Psychotherapy can help you rethink these issues and find purpose and identity in new ways.

Modulating Activity Levels and Self-Care

Some people with FM and CFS get scared of being active, because the pain and fatigue of doing too much feels like a punishment. As a result, they may actually withdraw from life more than is necessary. Psychotherapy can help you gain the courage and self-awareness you need to find just the right level of physical activity. Psychotherapy can also help you learn to pace yourself as you begin to have better days, so that you don't overdo.

Most people who recover from FM and CFS make fairly far-reaching changes in their self-care behavior. This tends to include being careful about what they eat, so that they only select foods that make them feel good and support their long-term health. However, food is central to many social relationships and this isn't the way most people eat. If you used to do most of your socializing with friends at restaurants, bars, or coffeehouses that don't serve the kind of foods and beverages that you now eat—or if your family or friends don't know how to cook the foods you need when you go to visit them—you may experience some very uncomfortable feelings about being different. And because your new ways of eating may unpleasantly challenge them to look at their own ways, friends and family may do subtle—or not-so-subtle—things that add to your discomfort. If you're to stick with eating foods you know are good for you, you'll have to renegotiate these food-related social interactions. Psychotherapy can help give you the conversation, assertiveness, and coping skills that you need—and help you stay focused on the value of taking care of yourself even when loved ones aren't as supportive as you'd like them to be.

Managing Your Health Care

When you become ill with FM or CFS, you may develop an urgent need to learn about your illness, make decisions, and solve problems, just when you're feeling your worst. It's easy to get overwhelmed and worry about your ability to make the best treatment decisions. Psychotherapy can help you sort it all out.

Issues may also arise in your relationships with your health care practitioners. When you're feeling very ill, you may also feel vulnerable and needy in your relationships with your practitioners. And because FM and CFS aren't well understood by some physicians, some may exhibit a dismissive or negative attitude toward you. Even with health care professionals who know how to help you, results may not come as quickly as you need them to; sometimes it's hard to know whether to continue to trust this health care provider and treatment, or try something new. You may need to acquire the ability to advocate for yourself. For example, if a health care practitioner explains something to you in terms that are hard to understand, you may need to ask for a simpler explanation. Similarly, sometimes there may be a need to educate a practitioner about a lab test, a supplement, or an off-label use of a drug. You have a right to dialogue with your health care practitioners and be actively involved in your care—even if practitioners aren't used to this.

Managing Your Pain

Pain that seems unmanageable can usually be influenced quite a bit by behavioral techniques. Our experience of pain can be changed by strategies such as activity pacing, distraction, relaxation techniques, hypnotherapy, etc. Psychotherapy can also help improve your sleep—and when your sleep is improved your pain may improve, and vice versa.

Finding a Psychotherapist

Sometimes it's hard to ask for help—especially if you're accustomed to being able to handle everything that comes your way. To make matters worse, there are still a lot of negative messages about psychotherapy in mainstream American culture. People from some cultures may not consider talking to a stranger as a valid way to solve emotional problems at all. But if psychotherapy does seem like a useful part of your overall health care plan, here are some guidelines for choosing a psychotherapist.

Psychotherapists generally have either a master's degree in counseling, social work, or marriage and family therapy, or a doctorate in counseling or clinical psychology. In all states, doctoral level psychologists are licensed. In some states, psychotherapists can be licensed with a master's degree and a certain amount of supervised clinical practice. A few psychiatrists—medical doctors who specialize in mental illnesses, usually through the use of medications—also do psychotherapy.

As with most health care practitioners, getting a referral from somebody you trust will help you feel confident that the person you've chosen is good at what they do. Your state or local psychology, counseling, or social work associations can provide referrals, too. If you have insurance coverage for mental health services, your insurance company will usually give you a list of people to choose from. If this is the case, the insurance company has already checked their credentials. If you get a referral from another source, check with the state agency that handles licensure to make sure that the person is licensed and hasn't had any disciplinary action taken against them.

When you first make telephone contact with potential psychotherapists, it's a good idea to ask them if they're familiar with FM and CFS. If they aren't but are willing to learn, they may still be an excellent choice—sharing this book with them can help them learn what they need to know. When you first meet with a psychotherapist, you can determine whether your personalities are a good match; it's best to trust your instincts on this. However, there may be times when a psychotherapist will ask difficult questions that bring up uncomfortable feelings. If you don't always feel completely relaxed and happy in your sessions, this may be for a reason other than a mismatch between you and the psychotherapist. When choosing a psychotherapist, ask yourself whether the psychotherapist is a person that you'll feel comfortable with while you experience uncomfortable emotions.

CHAPTER 13

Ayurvedic Medicine

Ayurveda is the ancient health care system of India. The term literally means the science of life, but ayurveda could be equally appropriately described as a science of balance. In ayurvedic philosophy, to achieve or maintain good health we must maintain balance between body, mind, and spirit, the different energies of which we are composed, and the use of our five senses. It's also crucial to maintain harmony with the natural elements, the seasons, and the principles—or natural laws—that govern how our bodies respond to outside influences.

Ayurveda is an all-encompassing health care system that addresses all fourteen of the elements of health; it doesn't need to be combined with other healing arts, although psychotherapy can be a helpful adjunctive treatment. Ayurveda may conflict with any approach that involves taking herbs.

The Five Elements

Central to ayurveda is the concept of five natural elements: ether, air, fire, water, and earth. Each part of the body is associated with one or more of these elements—e.g., fire is associated with the digestive tract, air with the lungs, etc. Each element also has an associated sense; for example, water is associated with the sense of taste and earth with the sense of smell. The five elements combine in pairs to form three basic energies, known as *doshas*. The balance of the elements determines how a dosha is expressed in a given individual.

The Three Doshas

The three doshas are *vata*, *pitta*, and *kapha*. Vata is a combination of ether and air, pitta is fire and water, and kapha is earth and water. All three doshas are in each of our bodies to varying degrees. Your own unique balance of doshas is called your *prakruti* or constitution. One dosha may dominate, two may share dominance, or all three may be equal. Your prakruti is determined at conception and doesn't change.

People with vata dominance tend to be thin, imaginative, quick moving, quick thinking, and have dry skin and hair. The qualities associated with vata are dry, cold, mobile, light, and rough. Pitta dominant people are strong, competitive, quick to anger, prone to skin irritations, and have good digestions and concentration. Pitta qualities are hot, light, sharp, mobile, and liquid. Kapha types are heavyset, slow, graceful, patient, loving, and prone to colds and respiratory allergies. The qualities associated with kapha are cold, moist, heavy, dense, dull, soft, and smooth.

Whatever your prakruti, the way to good health lies in balancing your doshas. When a dosha becomes too extreme, treatment aims to bring it back into harmony with the others—otherwise illness is likely to result; imbalances are called *vikruti*. Although the goal is to balance your doshas, the balance sought is the one that's uniquely your own, not the equal expression of all three doshas. It's a matter of optimizing your inborn constitution.

Everything we do has the potential to restore, maintain, or damage health. If we have an excess in one dosha and engage in lifestyle behaviors that further increase that dosha, those behaviors can damage our health. For example, if you have excess pitta, hot climates and eating spicy foods can aggravate this excess. If you have excess vata, an erratic lifestyle and eating cold, dry foods can be problematic. Careful attention must be given to daily lifestyle choices to avoid damage and maximize health.

Ayurvedic View of FM and CFS

In the ayurvedic view, FM and CFS are primarily seen as related to aggravated vata, accumulation of *ama* (toxins), and low *ojas* (immunity). It's believed a buildup of ama affects nerve function, causing pain and hypersensitivity to stimuli. Aggravated vata and accumulated ama also block the body's normal routes of detoxification. Another important factor in the ayurvedic view of FM and CFS is improper daily routines, including irregular mealtimes and bedtimes and extreme emotions and thoughts.

Ayurvedic Treatment

The following are some of the treatment techniques used to bring the doshas into balance; however, you should know that the very word "treatment" indicates a worldview quite different from that of ayurveda—in ayurveda the ways of harmonizing the doshas are simply ways of living rather than treatments for illness.

Five Sense Therapies

In ayurveda the five senses are seen as five opportunities to achieve balance. The sense of taste comes into play with dietary recommendations and herbs. Because foods share the same qualities of the doshas that our bodies do, dietary choices are a very important aspect of achieving optimal health. Foods must not only be good-tasting, fresh, nourishing, cooked with caring, and a delight to the eyes and the nose, they must also be balanced in terms of the different elements of taste: sweet, sour, astringent, salty, pungent, and bitter. Depending on your vikruti (imbalance), specific foods will be recommended, either to eat or avoid. Temperature of foods is also important and care is taken in combining foods in a given meal. Meals should be eaten while calm, in pleasant surroundings. According to Arora and Kumar (2003), digestive problems and resulting food allergies and sensitivities—common in FM and CFS—can be due to eating foods inappropriate for a person's prakruti.

Ayurvedic herbalism is a complex, highly developed art that also works with the sense of taste. In recent years, scientific research has found many of the herbs used in ayurveda effective for the symptoms they've traditionally been used to treat. For example, a study done by Bagul, Kanaki, and Rajani in 2005 showed that two ayurvedic herbal formulas had significant free radical scavenging qualities. And in reviewing the research on an ayurvedic herb called *bacopa*, Kidd (1999) found that bacopa shows beneficial effects for improving cognitive function and reducing anxiety, insomnia, headaches, and irritability.

There have, however, been some reports of ayurvedic herbal preparations containing lead or mercury, so it's important to be sure you purchase your herbs from a reputable source; your ayurvedic practitioner can help you find these sources. Keep in mind, too, that like any herbs, ayurvedic herbs can interact with prescription medications; it's best to consult an interaction database before combining herbs and medications.

In ayurveda the sense of touch is utilized through two kinds of bodywork: *abhyanga*—a massage with warm oil and long, soothing strokes, often recommended as a daily practice just before bathing; and *marma* therapy—rubbing points on the body where *prana*, or life energy, comes close to the surface and can be stimulated, sometimes with the use of sesame or other oils. This can be done by a trained marma therapist; in some cases, you can do it yourself.

According to ayurvedic principles, it's also important to surround yourself with things that please the eye, thus using vision as a means for healing. Particular emphasis is placed on colors—colors have qualities that relate to the doshas and the body's *chakras*, or energy centers. For example, surrounding yourself with the color orange can help alleviate aggravated vata.

The sense of smell is another channel for achieving balance. Specific essential oil scents, selected for your prakruti and vikruti, are used in massage, bathing, skin and hair care, or in a diffuser. The sense of hearing can be utilized to achieve balance through the use of chanting and *mantras*—specific words or sounds repeated while meditating.

Lifestyle

In ayurveda, yoga, meditation, and breathing practices are very important. The beneficial health effects of yoga are due to the ways the body positions, called *asanas*, stimulate the marma points. Depending on what your body needs, specific asanas may be prescribed. Yoga is often recommended for people with FM or CFS because of its stress-reducing qualities and the balance and healing it brings to the body. Asanas may need to be modified for people with FM. Many studies have shown that yoga can have a significant positive impact on a variety of health problems, including symptoms seen in FM and CFS (e.g., Manjunath and Telles 2005).

In ayurvedic philosophy, there isn't a clear distinction between the physical, emotional, and spiritual. All three are aspects of the life force.

So, although Western cultures tend to consider meditation as either a relaxation technique or a religious practice, in ayurveda, it's a spiritual practice that addresses the physical and the emotional as well. By meditating, we engage our own self-healing abilities. The effectiveness of meditation for stress reduction is well documented; because FM and CFS are stress-related illnesses, meditation is an important treatment tool.

Prana, or life energy, is best expressed in our breath. By balancing our breathing, we optimize our life energy. Ayurvedic practice includes a number of specific breathing exercises, called *pranayama*. These are often used just before meditating or just after performing yoga asanas.

Cleansing

In the ayurvedic view, a primary cause of unbalanced doshas is the buildup of ama—toxins caused by poor diet, extreme thoughts and emotions, improper lifestyle, external trauma, or spiritual influences. Ama can be eliminated through three channels, called *malas*: sweat, feces, and urine. A number of rituals optimize ama elimination through these channels. To people raised in Western nations, some of these practices can seem somewhat gruesome; in ayurveda, these practices are seen as an important part of health, well-being, and—through interconnectedness—spiritual attainment. Because ama buildup and digestion impairments are seen as central causes of FM and CFS, cleansing techniques are often used in treatments.

Preparatory Techniques (Purva Karma)

Snehan is the use of medicated oils for massage; sometimes the oils are ingested as well. *Swedana* is the use of heat for steam baths, poultices, and the application of warmed oils and other substances to the skin. Both techniques are believed to loosen the ama up and make it easier to expel.

Detoxification (Panchakarma)

There are five basic kinds of panchakarma: *vamana*, the use of emetics (substances that induce vomiting); *virecana*, the use of laxatives; *basti*, the use of enemas; *nasya*, nasal cleansing or the administration of herbal medicines or oils in liquid or vapor form through the nostrils; and *rakta mokshana*, bloodletting—usually accomplished nowadays by donating blood to a blood bank.

Follow-Up Techniques (Paschat Karma)

After the ama has been cleared from the body, specific diet and lifestyle recommendations will be made, called *samsarjan karma*, that aim to restore strength—particularly that of the digestive system, which can be weakened by the panchakarma.

How to Find an Ayurvedic Practitioner

In the U.S., ayurvedic practitioners aren't yet licensed. Although the National Ayurvedic Medical Association maintains guidelines for ayurvedic educational programs, these aren't recognized by state licensing boards. In some cases, an ayurvedic practitioner may have a license to practice another health profession—such as nursing, chiropractic, or physical therapy—however, there are also many ayurvedic practitioners who have no license but are equally well trained. See the Resources section at the back of this book for organizations that can provide you with names of ayurvedic practitioners in your area.

Your first ayurvedic session can last an hour or more, with shorter follow-up sessions. The ayurvedic physician will determine your prakruti and vikruti by asking you questions about your history, lifestyle, and preferences. He or she will make careful observations of your eyes, voice, nails, face, and posture and examine your tongue and pulse. There may also be forms and questionnaires to fill out. The goal is to develop a treatment plan that will combine the techniques described above to harmonize your own unique balance of doshas.

CHAPTER 14

Adjunctive and Emerging Approaches

In this book I've laid out the best of our current knowledge about what causes FM and CFS, why it's sometimes hard to get effective treatment, and how to orchestrate your own health care. I've also described a wide range of leading mainstream and alternative treatments; there are many viable options here, in many cases well-supported by research. You now have the information you need to make good health care decisions for yourself. I hope that you are beginning to develop a treatment plan specific to your needs—and that you'll soon feel good again!

In addition to the healing practices covered in chapters 4 through 13, you may hear about a number of other approaches, some of which are new and some of which are best used as adjuncts to other more comprehensive treatments. I've included many of them here to help you decide whether you want to explore them in more depth.

Adjunctive Approaches

In chapter 3 we discussed the importance of orchestrating health care to address all of the elements of health that are problematic for you. Most of the healing modalities we've discussed so far are like the string, brass, and woodwind sections of the orchestra: although the orchestra can't do without them, these instruments can stand alone and still make beautiful music. The approaches in this section are more like the cymbals or the triangle: they add to the sound of the orchestra, but you probably wouldn't want to hear them play a whole song by themselves. Although these approaches may be useful parts of your health care plan, because they only address a few elements of health—or address several of them in an incomplete way—they probably wouldn't be effective as a total health care plan.

Aromatherapy

Aromatherapy is based on the idea that inhaling scents can affect us physiologically. Essential oils—purified aromatic oils from various plants—are either diffused and then inhaled or inhaled during a bath or massage. Aromatherapy is particularly useful for emotional issues, and is said to enhance immunity, heal infections, improve breathing, overcome sleep problems, relieve pain, and treat many other medical conditions.

Biofeedback

In biofeedback, an external signal—typically a sound or a picture on a computer screen—is used to inform you about what's going on inside your body, so that you can voluntarily control processes such as heart rate and muscle tension. It's usually used for stress management and can be quite effective. It has also been used to control pain. Because stress is central to FM and CFS, using biofeedback to manage stress can have a beneficial effect on other elements of health as well.

Another form of biofeedback that's emerging as a possible treatment for FM and CFS—as well as a number of other conditions—is *electro-encephalogram (EEG)* biofeedback. With this approach, you get external feedback about the state of your brain waves. Voluntary control of brain waves is usually more difficult to attain, but research suggests it may help such FM- and CFS-related conditions as sleep problems, mood disorders, and pain; real-time brain imaging techniques hold promise for further developments in this area.

Flower Essences

Flower essence therapy is similar to homeopathy in that extremely dilute medicines are believed to have effects on the body much greater than would normally be expected. In this case, it's believed that certain supportive qualities that can positively impact people are embodied in flowers. The unique qualities and effects of flowers have been studied and catalogued so that flower essences can be selected to match the problem a person is trying to address. Generally, flower essences are most effective for spiritual and emotional concerns, but may indirectly affect other elements of health as well.

Shamanism and Spirituality

Since the beginning of time people have turned to spiritual healers for help, not just with spiritual problems, but with physical and emotional ones as well. A shaman would assist individuals both through prayer and ritual and by harnessing the supportive elements of community. Native traditions in nearly every part of the world still support practicing shamans; people can also create their own prayer-based health care support through friends or clergy. While the main element of health affected by shamanism is spirituality, other elements can be affected by this—and other spiritual practices—indirectly.

Balneotherapy

For centuries soaking in hot or cold water has been believed to have healing properties. The water might be spring water, mineral water, or herbalized water. It's believed that balneotherapy heals by stimulating circulation of blood and lymphatic fluid, relieving stress and tension, detoxifying, raising the body temperature to discourage viruses and bacteria, and through the absorption of minerals from the water. Balneotherapy can include taking mud baths, inhaling water vapor, and drinking mineral water. *Hydrotherapy* is the use of physical therapy techniques while a patient is immersed in water.

Emerging Approaches

The healing methods in this section don't have much—or in some cases, any—research support, although some people are using them for FM and CFS. However, every healing approach begins this way; it's only over time that it becomes possible to tell whether an approach has value. It would be a mistake to dismiss an approach just because it doesn't have a long history of supporting research or empirical evidence. It's important, though, to proceed with extreme caution with emerging healing methods; until they've stood the test of time, there isn't enough information available to know whether they're safe or effective. For all of the approaches described below, you'd do well to learn a lot more before deciding to incorporate them into your health care regimen. For some, a wait-and-see approach may be best.

Light Therapy

Light therapy encompasses a few different healing approaches that involve light. One is the use of bright lights to fight the effects of *seasonal affective disorder*—depression that strikes during the time of year when there is less natural light. A considerable amount of research supports bright light therapy for depression. There's also some support for its use with fatigue and sleep disorders, so it may be useful for FM and CFS. Another application of light for healing is *low level laser therapy* (LLLT), also called cold laser therapy. LLLT is the focused application of the cool end of the light spectrum. It's being used for pain, wound healing, and other health conditions. It's said to increase production of ATP, the energy currency used by our muscles.

Nutrigenomics

Genes are involved in many aspects of health—e.g., the use of nutrients, detoxification, organ function, hormone levels, etc. Scientists are now starting to explore the ways that subtle genetic differences can affect our health within a normal range of functioning. Knowing the variations in your genetic endowment may help you make wise lifestyle choices—for example, about food that will enhance your health. Given that recent research findings indicate family patterns in the incidence of FM and CFS, this approach may be useful for those with these conditions.

Intravenous Micronutrient Therapy

In *intravenous micronutrient therapy*, vitamins and minerals are administered through an intravenous drip, to deliver higher doses and bypass the digestive process. One formula that has been used with FM and CFS is the *Myers' cocktail* (Gaby 2002).

Oxygenation Therapies

Because oxygen is needed for proper functioning of every aspect of our bodies, a number of technologies have been proposed to increase oxygen supply. It's said that these help with pain, fatigue, detoxification, fighting fungal overgrowth, and increasing immunity. Oxygen—or in some cases, hydrogen peroxide or ozone—is delivered by a number of methods, including inhalation, pressurized chambers, ozone steam baths, introduction into the nose or rectum, infusion into the blood, and oral ingestion. Throughout history various breathing techniques have also been used by different cultures to increase oxygen supply to tissue.

Cleansing Approaches

Because the buildup of toxins in the body is believed to be the source of a number of health problems, several techniques have been developed to clean toxins out of the body:

Colon Hydrotherapy

Colon hydrotherapy is the cleansing of the bowel to lighten the toxic load on the body, and free up the colon for more efficient function.

Far Infrared Sauna

Far infrared saunas are used to raise the body temperature to a level that's inhospitable to viruses and bacteria. This type of heat warms the body without warming the air—making it easier for us to tolerate—and promotes efficient sweating and detoxification.

Chelation Therapy

Chelation therapy is the injection or ingestion of substances that chemically bind with certain toxins—particularly heavy metals—to remove them from the body more easily. Already approved for use with lead poisoning and heart disease, chelation therapy is now being tried for FM and CFS.

Ultraviolet Blood Irradiation Therapy

Ultraviolet light has long been used to sterilize surgical instruments; it's now also being used to cleanse the blood of toxins and infections and stimulate the immune system. In *ultraviolet blood irradiation therapy* a small amount of blood is removed from the body, treated with ultraviolet light, and then returned.

Electrical Stimulation

Various electrical stimulation techniques have been used to manage the pain and other symptoms of FM and CFS. The most widely used one is *transcutaneous electrical nerve stimulation* (TENS), which has been used for pain management in mainstream medical settings; TENS involves applying low-voltage electricity to the site of pain in an effort to either stimulate endorphin release or scramble pain signals. Newer methods include *electrical twitch obtaining intramuscular stimulation* (ETOIMS), which involves inserting a thin needle where muscles meet nerves and applying low-voltage electricity, causing muscles to twitch, eventually relaxing them; *microcurrent stimulation*, which applies a current to trigger points; and *cranial electrotherapy stimulation*, which applies a similar current to the head and aims to improve mood as well as pain.

Note that for some people, health seems to be compromised by exposure to the electromagnetic radiation that leaks from appliances, electronic equipment, and electrical outlets. These effects can, however, be neutralized, which sometimes helps restore health.

Marshall Protocol

The *Marshall protocol* is a method for treating certain kinds of resistant bacterial infections. It involves taking a medication called Benicar in combination with a strict avoidance of sunlight, bright light, and vitamin-D-containing foods. Originally developed for a condition called sarcoidosis, the Marshall protocol is now being tried for FM and CFS.

Prolotherapy (Sclerotherapy)

In *prolotherapy* a sugar solution is injected into ligaments or tendons where they connect to bones, with the goal of causing local inflammations that will increase blood supply, bringing increased nutrients to the areas and stimulating the tissue to heal.

Low Frequency Sound Therapy (Infrasonic Therapy)

Low frequency sound waves are thought to be healing; *low frequency sound therapy* involves applying sound waves similar to ultrasound to the body, either through the use of a small portable device or through a specially designed chair that usually also incorporates massage. It's thought that this relieves pain and promotes healing by stimulating cellular repair.

Pet Therapy

Since laughter has healing powers of its own, I'll end this final chapter with one of the most unusual and amusing approaches to treating pain I've ever encountered. A breed of dog called Mexican Hairless, or Xolo, is used to apply healing warmth to areas of pain. Apparently because these dogs are hairless, they generate more than the usual amount of body heat and are, quite literally, "hot dogs."

Resources

Acufinder.com—referrals to acupuncturists in your area. www.acu
finder.com

Acupuncture.com—explains the principles behind TCM and provides
research findings. www.acupuncture.com

American Botanical Council—membership fee gives access to online
Commission E monographs. www.herbalgram.org

American Herbalists Guild—directory of practitioners. www.ameri
canherbalistsguild.com

American Psychological Association—information about mental illness
and psychotherapy. www.apa.org

Association of State and Provincial Psychology Boards—information
about psychotherapy plus contact information for state boards regulating psychologists. www.asppb.org

Basch, E., and C. Ulbricht. 2004. *Natural Standard Herb and Supplement
Handbook: The Clinical Bottom Line.* St. Louis, MO: Mosby.

Bastyr University—naturopath referral network, plus useful library
resources. www.bastyr.edu

California College of Ayurveda—research and background articles
plus referrals to certified ayurvedic clinicians. www.ayurvedacollege
.com

Center for Science in the Public Interest's Guide to Food Additives. www.cspinet.org/reports/chemcuisine.htm

CFS Computational Challenge (C³)—a collection of studies of the genetics underlying CFS; results published in the April 2006 issue of the journal *Pharmacogenomics*. *Pharmacogenomics*' Web site: www .futuremedicine.com. Press release about C³: www.cfids.org/advo cacy/2006/pharma.pdf

Food elimination diets—information about identifying food sensitivities. www.foodintol.com

HealingFoodReference.com—listings of foods, herbs, and supplements that can be used to treat illness and related research citations; associated Web sites have news about natural health. www.healing foodreference.com

HerbMed—searchable online herbal database (nominal daily subscription fee). www.herbmed.org

International Bibliographic Information on Dietary Supplements (IBIDS)—extensive database of published articles, run under the auspices of the National Institutes of Health. http://grande.nal.usda .gov/ibids/index.php

International College of Applied Kinesiology—information about AK, including research abstracts and a directory of qualified professionals. www.icakusa.com

Journal of Alternative and Complementary Medicine—special issue on homeopathy, volume 11(5), October 2005; full text available at the journal's Web site (no charge). www.liebertonline.com/toc/acm/11/5

Mobility Limited—gentle exercise videos suitable for people with FM or CFS (retailer). www.mobilityltd.com

National Ayurvedic Medical Association—standards for ayurvedic educational programs. www.ayurveda-nama.org

National Certification Board for Therapeutic Massage and Bodywork—referrals to certified massage therapists and other information. 1-800-296-0664 or www.nctmb.com

National Certification Commission for Acupuncture and Oriental Medicine—national credentialing services; maintains an online directory of practitioners. www.nccaom.org

National Institute of Ayurvedic Medicine—referrals to ayurvedic practitioners. www.niam.com

Physicians' Desk Reference (PDR)—free searchable herbal database. www.pdrhealth.com/drug_info/index.html

Phytotherapy Research Labs—referrals to herbalists who use high quality herbal products. 1-931-593-3780

The Council for Homeopathic Certification—credentialing services; maintains an online directory of qualified homeopaths. www.homeo pathicdirectory.com

The Longwood Herbal Task Force—monographs on herbs, including research citations. www.longwoodherbal.org

The National Center for Homeopathy—many useful resources, including articles on homeopathy and referrals to practicing homeopaths. www.homeopathic.org

Touch Research Institute—summaries of research findings on massage therapy. www.miami.edu/touch-research/about.htm

United Plant Savers—an organization devoted to preserving supplies of native healing plants. www.unitedplantsavers.org

University of Maryland Medical Center's Center for Integrative Medicine—summarizes the theory of ayurveda and includes a bibliography of research articles. www.umm.edu/altmed/ConsModalities/Ayurvedacm.html

References

Abraham, G., and J. Flechas. 1992. Management of fibromyalgia: Rationale for the use of magnesium and malic acid. *Journal of Nutritional Medicine* 3:49-59.

Alexander, R., L. Bradley, G. Alarcon, M. Triana-Alexander, L. Aaron, K. Alberts, M. Martin, and K. Stewart. 1998. Sexual and physical abuse in women with fibromyalgia: Association with outpatient health care utilization and pain medication usage. *Arthritis Care and Research* 11:102-115.

Ali, M. 2003. The cause of fibromyalgia: The respiratory-to-fermentative shift (the Dysox state) in ATP production. *Journal of Integrative Medicine* 8:-140.

Allen, L. A., J. I. Escobar, P. M. Lehrer, M. A. Gara, and R. L. Woolfolk. 2002. Psychosocial treatments for multiple unexplained physical symptoms: A review of the literature. *Psychosomatic Medicine* 64:939-950.

Allen, R., P. M. Becker, R. Bogan, M. Schmidt, C. A. Kushida, J. M. Fry, J. S. Poceta, and D. Winslow. 2004. Ropinirole decreases periodic leg movements and improves sleep parameters in patients with restless legs syndrome. *Sleep* 27(5):907-914.

Alvarez, L. B., J. L. Alonso Valdivielso, J. Alegre Lopez, C. Martel Soteres, J. L. Viejo Banuelos, and A. Maranon Cabello. 1996. Fibromyalgia syndrome: Overnight falls in arterial oxygen saturation. *American Journal of Medicine* 101(1):54-60.

Ames, B. N. 2003. The metabolic tune-up: Metabolic harmony and disease prevention. *Journal of Nutrition* 133(5 Suppl.): 1544S-1548S.

Anderson, R. 1994. *Stress Effects on Chromium Nutrition in Humans and Animals.* 10th ed. Nottingham, UK: Nottingham University Press.

Anderson, R. A. 1997. Nutritional factors influencing the glucose/insulin system: Chromium. *Journal of the American College of Nutrition* 16(5):404-410.

Appleton, N. 1996. *Lick the Sugar Habit.* New York: Avery Publishing Group.

Arora, D., and M. Kumar. 2003. Food allergies—leads from Ayurveda. *Indian Journal of Medical Science* 57:57-63.

Avraham, Y., S. Hao, S. Mendelson, and E. M. Berry. 2001. Tyrosine improves appetite, cognition, and exercise tolerance in activity anorexia. *Medicine and Science in Sports and Exercise* 33(12):2104-2110.

Axe, E. K., P. Satz, N. L. Rasgon, and F. I. Fawzy. 2004. Major depressive disorder in chronic fatigue syndrome: A CDC surveillance study. *Journal of Chronic Fatigue Syndrome* 12(3):7-23.

Badawy, A. A., C. J. Morgan, M. B. Llewelyn, S. R. Albuquerque, and A. Farmer. 2005. Heterogeneity of serum tryptophan concentration and availability to the brain in patients with the chronic fatigue syndrome. *Journal of Psychopharmacology* 19(4):385-391.

Bagis, S., L. Tamer, G. Sahin, R. Bilgin, H. Guler, B. Ercan, and C. Erdogan. 2005. Free radicals and antioxidants in primary fibromyalgia: An oxidative stress disorder? *Rheumatology International* 25(3):188-190.

Bagul, M., N. Kanaki, and M. Rajani. 2005. Evaluation of free radical scavenging properties of two classical polyherbal formulations. *Indian Journal of Experimental Biology* 43(8):732-736.

Baraniuk, J. N., B. Casado, H. Maibach, D. J. Clauw, L. K. Pannell, and S. Hess. 2005. A chronic fatigue syndrome-related proteome in human cerebrospinal fluid. *BioMed Central Neurology* 5:22.

Baseman, J. B., and J. G. Tully. 1997. Mycoplasmas: Sophisticated, reemerging, and burdened by their notoriety. *Emerging Infectious Diseases* 1(3):21-32.

Bates, D. W., D. Buchwald, J. Lee, P. Kith, T. Doolittle, C. Rutherford, W. H. Churchill, P. H. Schur, M. Wener, D. Wybenga, et al. 1995. Clinical laboratory test findings in patients with chronic fatigue syndrome. *Archives of Internal Medicine* 155(1):97-103.

Beck, M. A., O. Levander, and J. Handy. 2003. Selenium deficiency and viral infection. *Journal of Nutrition* 133:1463S-1467S.

Bennett, A. L., D. M. Mayes, L. R. Fagioli, R. Guerriero, and A. L. Komaroff. 1997. Somatomedin C (insulin-like growth factor I) levels in patients with chronic fatigue syndrome. *Journal of Psychiatric Research* 31(1):91-96.

Benton, D., and R. Cook. 1991. The impact of selenium supplementation on mood. *Biological Psychiatry* 29(11):1092-1098.

Benton, D., and R. T. Donohoe. 1999. The effects of nutrients on mood. *Public Health Nutrition* 2(3A):403-409.

Benzel, E., S. Sridharan, A. A. Krishnaney, A. Henwood, and W. S. Wilke. 2005. Chiari malformation and fibromyalgia. *Spine Universe* (originally published 9/5/2002, updated 7/6/2005). http://www. spineuniverse.com/displayarticle.php/article1884.html (accessed July 8, 2006).

Berg, D., L. H. Berg, J. Couvaras, and H. Harrison. 1999. Chronic fatigue syndrome and/or fibromyalgia as a variation of antiphospholipid antibody syndrome: An explanatory model and approach to laboratory diagnosis. *Blood Coagulation and Fibrinolysis* 10(7):435-438.

Berman, B., J. Ezzo, V. Hadhazy, and J. Swyers. 1999. Is acupuncture effective in the treatment of fibromyalgia? *Journal of Family Practice* 48(3):213-218.

Biancalana, M. Questions and answers with Mary Biancalana, CMTPT. Posture Dynamics Web site. http://www4.adhost.com /posturedyn/qna/biancalana.html (accessed July 14, 2006).

Birdsall, T. C. 1998. 5-Hydroxytryptophan: A clinically-effective serotonin precursor. *Alternative Medicine Review* 3(4):271-280.

Blanco, L. E., F. J. de Serres, E. Fernandez-Bustillo, D. A. Kassam, D. Arbesu, C. Rodriguez, and J. C. Torre. 2005. Alpha1-Antitrypsin and fibromyalgia: New data in favour of the inflammatory hypothesis of fibromyalgia. *Medical Hypotheses* 64(4):759-769.

Blumenthal, M., and W. Busse, eds. 1998. *The Complete German Commission E Monographs: Therapeutic Guide to Herbal Medicines.* New York: Lippincott, Williams & Wilkins.

Bounous, G., and J. Molson. 1999. Competition for glutathione precursors between the immune system and the skeletal muscle: Pathogenesis of chronic fatigue syndrome. *Medical Hypotheses* 53(4):347-349.

Bower, J., M. Kemeny, S. Taylor, and J. Fahey. 2003. Finding positive meaning and its association with natural killer cell cytotoxicity among participants in a bereavement-related disclosure intervention. *Annals of Behavioral Medicine* 25(2):146-155.

Bressa, G. M. 1994. S-adenosyl-l-methionine (SAMe) as antidepressant: Meta-analysis of clinical studies. *Acta Neurologica Scandinavica Supplementum* 154:7–14.

Brzezinski, A. 1997. Melatonin in humans. *New England Journal of Medicine* 336(3):186-195.

Buchwald, D., J. Umali, and M. Stene. 1996. Insulin-like growth factor-I (somatomedin C) levels in chronic fatigue syndrome and fibromyalgia. *Journal of Rheumatology* 23(4):739-742.

Buchwald, D., M. Wener, T. Pearlman, and P. Kith. 1997. Markers of inflammation and immune activation in chronic fatigue and chronic fatigue syndrome. *Journal of Rheumatology* 24(2): 372-376.

Buskila, D., and L. Neumann. 2005. Genetics of fibromyalgia. *Current Pain and Headache Reports* 9(5):313-315.

Buskila, D., L. Neumann, G. Vaisberg, D. Alkalay, and F. Wolfe. 1997. Increased rates of fibromyalgia following cervical spine injury: A controlled study of 161 cases of traumatic injury. *Arthritis & Rheumatism* 40(3):446-452.

Cantorna, M. T., Y. Zhu, M. Froicu, and A. Wittke. 2004. Vitamin D status, 1,25-dihydroxyvitamin D_3, and the immune system. *American Journal of Clinical Nutrition* 80(6):1717S-1720S.

Caruso, I., P. P. Sarzi, M. Cazzola, and V. Azzolini. 1990. Double-blind study of 5-hydroxytryptophan versus placebo in the treatment of primary fibromyalgia syndrome. *Journal of International Medical Research* 18:201-209.

Cassar, M. P. 1999. Massage for detoxification. Adapted from *Handbook of Massage Therapy: A Complete Guide for the Student and Professional Massage Therapist*. Oxford: Butterworth-Heinemann; 1999. http://www.positivehealth.com/permit/Articles/Massage/cassar 39.htm (accessed June 5, 2006).

Ciccone, D. S., D. Elliott, H. Chandler, S. Nayak, and K. Raphael. 2005. Sexual and physical abuse in women with fibromyalgia syndrome: A test of the trauma hypothesis. *Clinical Journal of Pain* 21(5):378-386.

Cleare, A. J., C. Messa, E. A. Rabiner, and P. M. Grasby. 2005. 5-HT(1A) receptor binding in chronic fatigue syndrome measured using positron emission tomography and [(11)C]WAY-100635. *Biological Psychiatry* 57(3):239-246.

Collinge, W. 1993. *Recovering from Chronic Fatigue Syndrome: A Guide to Self-Empowerment.* London: Putnam/Perigree.

Conklin, S. 2006. Abstract of paper presented at the 2006 Annual Scientific Meeting of the American Psychosomatic Society, Denver, CO, March 1-4. http://www.eurekalert.org/pub_releases/2006-03/uopm-o3f022706.php (accessed July 3, 2006).

Connor, J. R., P. J. Boyer, S. L. Menzies, B. Dellinger, R. P. Allen, W. G. Ondo, and C. J. Earley. 2003. Neuropathological examination suggests impaired brain iron acquisition in restless legs syndrome. *Neurology* 61:304–309.

Connor, T. J., and B. Leonard. 1998. Depression, stress, and immunological activation: The role of cytokines in depressive disorders. *Life Sciences* 62:583-606.

Cox, I., M. Campbell, and D. Dowson. 1991. Red blood cell magnesium and chronic fatigue syndrome. *Lancet* 337(8744):757-760.

Crook, W. 1999. *The Yeast Connection Handbook.* Jackson, TN: Professional Books.

Cutler, E. 2003. *The Food Allergy Cure: A New Solution to Food Cravings, Obesity, Depression, Headaches, Arthritis, and Fatigue.* New York: Three Rivers Press.

De Becker, P., K. De Meirleir, E. Joos, I. Campine, E. Van Steenberge, J. Smitz, and B. Velkeniers. 1999. Dehydroepiandrosterone (DHEA) response to i.v. ACTH in patients with chronic fatigue syndrome. *Hormone and Metabolic Research* 31(1):18-21.

De Civita, J., S. Bernatsky, and P. Dobkin. 2004. The role of depression in mediating the association between sexual abuse history and pain in women with fibromyalgia. *Psychology, Health & Medicine* 9(4):450-455.

Deijen, J. B., C. J. Wientjes, H. F. Vullinghs, P. A. Cloin, and J. J. Langefeld. 1999. Tyrosine improves cognitive performance and reduces blood pressure in cadets after one week of a combat training course. *Brain Research Bulletin* 48(2):203-209.

de Lange, F. P., J. Kalkman, G. Bleijenberg, P. Hagoort, J. van der Meer, and I. Toni. 2005. Gray matter volume reduction in the chronic fatigue syndrome. *Neuroimage* 26(3):777-781.

Deluze, C., L. Bosia, A. Zirbs, A. Chantraine, and T. L. Vischer. 1992. Electroacupuncture in fibromyalgia: Results of a controlled trial. *British Medical Journal* 305(6864):1249-1252.

Diego, M., T. Fied, C. Sanders, and M. Hernandez-Reif. 2004. Massage therapy of moderate and light pressure and vibrator effects on EEG and heart rate. *International Journal of Neuroscience* 114(1):31-44.

Di Giorgio, A., M. Hudson, W. Jerjes, and A. J. Cleare. 2005. 24-hour pituitary and adrenal hormone profiles in chronic fatigue syndrome. *Psychosomatic Medicine* 67(3):433-440.

Droge, W., and E. Holm. 1997. Role of cysteine and glutathione in HIV infection and other diseases associated with muscle wasting and immunological dysfunction. *FASEB Journal* 11(13):1077-1089. http://www.fasebj.org/cgi/reprint/11/13/1077 (accessed June 21, 2006).

Dunstan, H. R., N. R. McGregor, H. L. Butt, T. K. Roberts, I. J. Klineberg, S. H. Niblett, T. Rothbirch, and I. Buttfield. 2000. Characterization of differential amino acid homeostasis amongst population subgroups: A basis for determining specific amino acid requirements. *Journal of Nutritional & Environmental Medicine* 10(3):211-223.

Eisinger, J. 1998. Alcohol, thiamin, and fibromyalgia. *Journal of the American College of Nutrition* 17(3):300–303.

Eisinger, J., A. Plantamura, P. Marie, and T. Ayavou. 1994. Selenium and magnesium status in fibromyalgia. *Magnesium Research* 7(3-4):285-288.

Elson, C. O., R. B. Sartor, S. R. Targan, and W. J. Sandborn. 2003. Challenges in IBD Research: Updating the scientific agendas. *Inflammatory Bowel Diseases* 9(3):137-153.

Elvin, A., A. K. Siosteen, A. Nilsson, and E. Kosek. 2006. Research: Decreased muscle blood flow in fibromyalgia patients during standardised muscle exercise. *European Journal of Pain* 10(2):137-144.

Eriksen, W. 2004. Linking work factors to neck myalgia: The nitric oxide/oxygen ratio hypothesis. *Medical Hypotheses* 62(5):721-726.

Farah, D. A., I. Calder, L. Benson, and J. Mackenzie. 1985. Specific food intolerance: Its place as a cause of gastrointestinal symptoms. *Gut* 26:164-168.

Feinstein, A. 1998. *Prevention's Healing with Vitamins*. Emmaus, PA: Rodale Books.

Fibromyalgia Network. 1995. Off-loading your symptoms: Why this might help and how to do it! *Fibromyalgia Network* newsletter. http://www.fmnetnews.com/pages/offload.html (accessed July 8, 2006).

Field, T., M. Diego, C. Cullen, M. Hernandez-Reif, W. Sunshine, and S. Douglas. 2002. Fibromyalgia pain and substance P decrease and sleep improves after massage therapy. *Journal of Clinical Rheumatology* 8(2):72-76.

Field, T., M. Hernandez-Reif, M. Diego, S. Schanberg, and C. Kuhn. 2005. Cortisol decreases and serotonin and dopamine increase following massage therapy. *International Journal of Neuroscience* 115(10):1397-1413.

Field, T., M. Hernandez-Reif, S. Hart, O. Quintino, L. Drose, T. Field, C. Kuhn, and S. Schanberg. 1997. Sexual abuse effects are lessened by massage therapy. *Journal of Bodywork and Movement Therapies* 1:65-69.

Field, T., G. Ironson, F. Scafidi, T. Nawrocki, A. Gonclaves, I. Burman, J. Pickens, N. Fox, S. Schanberg, and C. Kuhn. 1996. Massage therapy reduces anxiety and enhances EEG pattern of alertness and math computations. *International Journal of Neuroscience* 86:197-205.

Forsyth, L. M., H. G. Preuss, A. L. MacDowell, L. Chiazze Jr., G. D. Birkmayer, and J. A. Bellanti. 1999. Therapeutic effects of oral NADH on the symptoms of patients with chronic fatigue syndrome. *Annals of Allergy, Asthma, and Immunology* 82(2):185-191.

Frustaci, A., N. Magnavita, C. Chimenti, M. Caldarulo, E. Sabbioni, R. Pietra, C. Cellini, G. F. Possati, and A. Maseri. 1999. Marked elevation of myocardial trace elements in idiopathic dilated cardiomyopathy compared with secondary cardiac dysfunction. *Journal of the American College of Cardiology* 33(6):1578-1583.

Fukuda, K., S. Straus, I. Hickie, M. Sharpe, J. Dobbins, A. Komaroff, and the International Chronic Fatigue Syndrome Study Group. 1994. The chronic fatigue syndrome: A comprehensive approach to its definition and study. *Annals of Internal Medicine* 121(12):953-959.

Fulle, S., P. Mecocci, G. Fano, I. Vecchiet, A. Vecchini, D. Racciotti, A. Cherubini, E. Pizzigallo, L. Vecchiet, U. Senin, and M. Beal. 2000. Specific oxidative alterations in vastus lateralis muscle of patients with the diagnosis of chronic fatigue syndrome. *Free Radical Biology and Medicine* 15:1252-1259.

Gaby, A. 2002. Intravenous nutrient therapy: The "Myers' cocktail." *Alternative Medicine Review* 7(5):389-403.

Galland, L. 1998. *Power Healing: Use the New Integrated Medicine to Cure Yourself.* New York: Random House.

Gardner, M. L. 1988. Gastrointestinal absorption of intact proteins. *Annual Review of Nutrition* 8:329-350.

Gebhart, B., and J. A. Jorgenson. 2004. Benefit of ribose in a patient with fibromyalgia. *Pharmacotherapy* 24(11):1646-1648.

Giesecke, T., R. Gracely, D. Williams, M. Geisser, F. Petzke, and D. Clauw. 2005. The relationship between depression, clinical pain, and experimental pain in a chronic pain cohort. *Arthritis & Rheumatism* 52(5):1577-1584.

Gold, A. R., F. Dipalo, M. Gold, and J. Broderick. 2004. Inspiratory airflow dynamics during sleep in women with fibromyalgia. *Sleep* 27:459-466.

Goldberg, B. 1998. *Chronic Fatigue, Fibromyalgia, and Environmental Illness.* Tiburon, CA: Future Medicine.

Goldenberg, D., C. Burckhardt, and L. Crofford. 2004. Management of fibromyalgia syndrome. *Journal of the American Medical Association* 292(19):2388-2395.

Goldstein, J. 1993. *Chronic Fatigue Syndromes: The Limbic Hypothesis.* Binghamton, NY: Haworth Medical Press.

Gordon, C., C. Emiliozzi, and M. Zartarian. 2006. Use of a mechanical massage technique in the treatment of fibromyalgia: A preliminary study. *Archives of Physical Medical Rehabilitation* 87(1):145-147.

Gracely, R. H., F. Petzke, J. M. Wolf, and D. J. Clauw. 2002. Functional magnetic resonance imaging evidence of augmented pain processing in fibromyalgia. *Arthritis & Rheumatism* 46(5):1333-1343.

Gray, J. B., and A. M. Martinovic. 1994. Eicosanoids and essential fatty acid modulation in chronic disease and the chronic fatigue syndrome. *Medical Hypotheses* 43:31-42.

Haas, E., and B. Levin. 2006. *Staying Healthy with Nutrition 21st Century Edition: The Complete Guide to Diet and Nutritional Medicine.* Berkeley, CA: Celestial Arts.

Hains, G., and F. Hains. 2000. A combined ischemic compression and spinal manipulation in the treatment of fibromyalgia: A preliminary estimate of dose and efficacy. *Journal of Manipulative Physiological Therapies* 23(4):225-230.

Hardeland, R. 2005. Antioxidative protection by melatonin: Multiplicity of mechanisms from radical detoxification to radical avoidance. *Endocrine* 27(2):119-130.

Heap, L. C., T. J. Peters, and S. Wessely. 1999. Vitamin B status in patients with chronic fatigue syndrome. *Journal of the Royal Society of Medicine* 92(4):183-185.

Heffez, D., R. Ross, Y. Shade-Zeldow, K. Kostas, S. Shah, R. Gottschalk, D. Elias, A. Shepard, S. Leurgans, and C. Moore. 2004. Clinical evidence for cervical myelopathy due to Chiari malformation and spinal stenosis in a non-randomized group of patients with the diagnosis of fibromyalgia. *European Spine Journal* 13(6):516-523.

Holick, M. F., and M. Jenkins. 2005. *The UV Advantage: The Medical Breakthrough That Shows How to Harness the Power of the Sun for Your Health.* New York: Simon & Schuster.

Hudson, J. I., D. L. Goldenberg, H. G. Pope Jr., P. E. Keck Jr., and L. Schlesinger. 1992. Comorbidity of fibromyalgia with medical and psychiatric disorders. *American Journal of Medicine* 92(4):363-367.

Jacobsen, S., B. Danneskiold-Samsoe, and R. B. Andersen. 1991. Oral S-adenosylmethionine in primary fibromyalgia. Double-blind clinical evaluation. *Scandinavian Journal of Rheumatology* 20:294-302.

Jacobson, W., T. Saich, L. K. Borysiewicz, W. M. Behan, P. O. Behan, and T. G. Wreghitt. 1993. Serum folate and chronic fatigue syndrome. *Neurology* 43(12):2645-2647.

Jammes, Y., J. Steinberg, O. Mambrini, F. Bregeon, and S. Delliaux. 2005. Chronic fatigue syndrome: Assessment of increased oxidative stress and altered muscle excitability in response to incremental exercise. *Journal of Internal Medicine* 257(3):299-310.

Jasmin, L., S. D. Rabkin, A. Granato, A. Boudah, and P. T. Ohara. 2003. Analgesia and hyperalgesia from GABA-mediated modulation of the cerebral cortex. *Nature* 424(6946):316-320.

Jefferies, W. 1994. Mild adrenocortical deficiency, chronic allergies, autoimmune disorders, and the chronic fatigue syndrome: A continuation of the cortisone story. *Medical Hypotheses* 42:183-189.

Juhl, J. H. 1998. Fibromyalgia and the serotonin pathway. *Alternative Medicine Review* 3(5):367-375.

Kaplan, M. 2001. Hypercoagulation: The CFS/FM plot thickens. *Carousel Network News* 8(5). http://www.anapsid.org/cnd/diffdx /hypercoagulation.html (accessed July 15, 2006).

Kaslow, J. E., L. Rucker, and R. Onishi. 1989. Liver extract-folic acid-cyanocobalamin vs. placebo for chronic fatigue syndrome. *Archives of Internal Medicine* 149:2501-2503.

Kaushik, N., D. Fear, S. Richards, C. McDermott, E. Nuwaysir, P. Kellam, T. Harrison, R. Wilkinson, D. Tyrrell, S. Holgate, and J. Kerr. 2005. Gene expression in peripheral blood mononuclear cells from patients with chronic fatigue syndrome. *Journal of Clinical Pathology* 58:826-832.

Kelly, G. 1997a. Hydrochloric acid: Physiological functions and clinical implications. *Alternative Medicine Review* 2(2):116-127.

———— 1997b. Sports nutrition: A review of selected nutritional supplements for bodybuilders and strength athletes. *Alternative Medicine Review* 2(3):184-201.

———— 1998. L-Carnitine: Therapeutic applications of a conditionally-essential amino acid. *Alternative Medicine Review* 3(5):345-360.

Kennedy, G., V. Spence, M. McLaren, A. Hill, C. Underwood, and J. J. Belch. 2005. Oxidative stress levels are raised in chronic fatigue syndrome and are associated with clinical symptoms. *Free Radical Biology and Medicine* 39(5):584-589.

Kidd, P. 1999. A review of nutrients and botanicals in the integrative management of cognitive dysfunction. *Alternative Medicine Review* 4(3):144-161.

————— 2005. Neurodegeneration from mitochondrial insufficiency: Nutrients, stem cells, growth factors, and prospects for brain rebuilding using integrative management. *Alternative Medicine Review* 10(4):268-293.

Kingsbury, K. J., L. Kay, and M. Hjelm. 1998. Contrasting plasma free amino acid patterns in elite athletes: Association with fatigue and infection. *British Journal of Sports Medicine* 32(1):25-32.

Kleijnen, J., P. Knipschild, and G. ter Riet. 1991. Clinical trials of homeopathy. *British Medical Journal* 302:316-323.

Knox, K. K., A. Cocchetto, E. Jordan, D. Leech, and D. R. Carrigan. 2004. Deficiency in the expression of stat1 protein in a subpopulation of patients with chronic fatigue syndrome (CFS). Paper presented at the AACFS Seventh International Conference, Madison, WI, October 8-10. http://www.ivpresearch.org/cfs _stat1_2004.htm (accessed July 15, 2006).

Kodama, M., T. Kodama, and M. Murakami. 1996. The value of the dehydroepiandrosterone-annexed vitamin C infusion treatment in the clinical control of chronic fatigue syndrome (CFS). II. Characterization of CFS patients with special reference to their response to a new vitamin C infusion treatment. *In Vivo* 10(6):585-596.

Korszun, A., L. Sackett-Lundeen, E. Papadopoulos, C. Brucksch, L. Masterson, N. C. Engelberg, E. Haus, M. A. Demitrack, and L. Crofford. 1999. Melatonin levels in women with fibromyalgia and chronic fatigue syndrome. *Journal of Rheumatology* 26(12):2675-2680.

Kozlovsky, K. S., P. B. Moser, S. Reiser, and R. A. Anderson. 1986. Effects of diets high in simple sugars on urinary chromium losses. *Metabolism* 35:515-518.

Kramis, R. C., W. Roberts, and R. Gillette. 1996. Non-nociceptive aspects of persistent musculoskeletal pain. *Journal of Orthopaedic and Sports Physical Therapy* 24(4):255-267.

Krotkiewski, M., M. Gudmundsson, P. Backström, and K. Mandroukas. 1982. Zinc and muscle strength and endurance. *Acta Physiologica Scandinavica* 116(3):309-311.

Kuratsune, H., K. Yamaguti, M. Sawada, S. Kodate, T. Machii, Y. Kanakura, and T. Kitani. 1998. Dehydroepiandrosterone sulfate deficiency in chronic fatigue syndrome. *International Journal of Molecular Medicine* 1(1):143-146.

Kwiatek, R., L. Barnden, R. Tedman, R. Jarrett, J. Chew, C. Rowe, and K. Pile. 2000. Regional cerebral blood flow in fibromyalgia: Single-photon-emission computed tomography evidence of reduction in the pontine tegmentum and thalami. *Arthritis & Rheumatism* 43(12):2823-2833.

Landis, C. A., M. J. Lentz, J. Tsuji, D. J. Buchwald, and L. F. Shaver. 2004. Pain, psychological variables, sleep quality, and natural killer cell activity in midlife women with and without fibromyalgia. *Brain, Behavior, and Immunity* 18(4):304-313.

Laske, C., E. Stransky, G. Eschweiler, R. Klein, A. Wittorf, T. Leyhe, E. Richartz, N. Kohler, M. Bartels, G. Buchkremer, and K. Schott. 2006. Increased BDNF serum concentration in fibromyalgia with or without depression or antidepressants. *Journal of Psychiatric Research* (April 3). http://www.ncbi.nlm.nih.gov /entrez/query.fcgi?db=pubmed&cmd=Retrieve&dopt=Abstract& list_uids=16600301&query_hl=6&itool=pubmed_docsum (accessed July 6, 2006).

Lee, J., J. Hanley, and V. Hopkins. 1999. *What Your Doctor May Not Tell You About Premenopause: Balance Your Hormones and Your Life from Thirty to Fifty*. New York: Warner Wellness.

Lentz, M. J., C. A. Landis, J. Rothermel, and J. L. Shaver. 1999. Effects of selective slow wave sleep disruption on musculoskeletal pain and fatigue in middle aged women. *Journal of Rheumatology* 26(7):1586-1592.

Linde, K., N. Clausius, G. Ramirez, D. Melchart, F. Eitel, L. Hedges, and W. Jonas. 1997. Are the clinical effects of homeopathy placebo effects? A meta-analysis of placebo-controlled trials. *Lancet* 350:834-843.

Liu, J., E. Head, A. M. Gharib, W. Yuan, R. T. Ingersoll, T. M. Hagen, C. W. Cotman, and B. N. Ames. 2002. Memory loss in old rats is associated with brain mitochondrial decay and RNA/DNA oxidation: Partial reversal by feeding acetyl-L-carnitine and/or R-α-lipoic acid. *Proceedings of the National Academy of Sciences of the United States of America* 99(4):2356–2361.

Logan, A. C., R. A. Venket, and D. Irani. 2003. Chronic fatigue syndrome: Lactic acid bacteria may be of therapeutic value. *Medical Hypotheses* 60(6):915-923.

Lowe, J. C. 2005. Air hunger to death: Breathing problems of hypothyroid patients (February 25). http://www.drlowe.com/jcl/comentry /breathingproblems.htm (accessed July 8, 2006).

Lucas, H., C. Brauch, L. Settas, and T. Theoharides. 2006. Fibromyalgia—new concepts of pathogenesis and treatment. *International Journal of Immunopathology and Pharmacology* 19(1):5-10.

Lund-Olesen, L. H., and K. Lund-Olesen. 1994. The etiology and possible treatment of chronic fatigue syndrome/fibromyalgia. *Medical Hypotheses* 43(1):55-58.

MacFarlane, J. G., B. Shahal, C. Mously, and H. Moldofsky. 1996. Periodic K-alpha sleep EEG activity and periodic limb movements during sleep: Comparisons of clinical features and sleep parameters. *Sleep* 19:200.

Maes, M., R. Verkerk, L. Delmeire, A. Van Gastel, F. van Hunsel, and S. Scharpe. 2000. Serotonergic markers and lowered plasma branched-chain-amino acid concentrations in fibromyalgia. *Psychiatry Research* 97(1):11-20.

Magaldi, M., L. Moltoni, G. Biasi, and R. Marcolongo. 2000. Changes in intracellular calcium and magnesium ions in the physiopathology of the fybromyalgia syndrome. *Minerva Medica* 91(7-8):137-140.

Maher, K. J., N. G. Klimas, and M. A. Fletcher. 2005. Chronic fatigue syndrome is associated with diminished intracellular perforin. *Clinical and Experimental Immunology* 142(3):505-511.

Malouf, R., and J. Grimley Evans. 2003. The effect of vitamin B_6 on cognition. *Cochrane Database of Systematic Reviews* (4):CD004393.

Manfredini, D., F. Tognini, G. Montagnani, L. Bazzichi, S. Bombardieri, and M. Bosco. 2004. Comparison of masticatory dysfunction in temporomandibular disorders and fibromyalgia. *Minerva Stomatologica* 53(11-12):641-650.

Manjunath, N., and S. Telles. 2005. Influence of yoga and ayurveda on self-rated sleep in a geriatric population. *Indian Journal of Medical Research* 121:683-690.

Martin, D. P., C. D. Sletten, B. A. Williams, and I. H. Berger. 2006. Improvement in fibromyalgia symptoms with acupuncture: Results of a randomized controlled trial. *Mayo Clinic Proceedings* 81(6):749-757.

Martinez-Lavin, M. 2004. Fibromyalgia as a sympathetically maintained pain syndrome. *Current Pain and Headache Reports* 8(5):385-389.

Mauskop, A., B. T. Altura, R. Q. Cracco, and B. M. Altura. 1996. Intravenous magnesium sulfate rapidly alleviates headaches of various types. *Headache* 36(3):154-160.

McBeth, J., Y. H. Chiu, A. J. Silman, D. Ray, R. Morriss, C. Dickens, A. Gupta, and G. J. Macfarlane. 2005. About somatizers: Fibromyalgia research: Hypothalamic-pituitary-adrenal stress axis function and the relationship with chronic widespread pain. *Arthritis Research and Therapy* 7(5):R992-R1000.

McLean, S. A., D. A. Williams, R. E. Harris, W. J. Kop, K. H. Groner, K. Ambrose, A. K. Lyden, R. H. Gracely, L. J. Crofford, M. E. Geisser, A. Sen, P. Biswas, and D. J. Clauw. 2005. Momentary relationship between cortisol secretion and symptoms in patients with fibromyalgia. *Arthritis & Rheumatism* 52(11):3660-3669.

Medical Economics, Joerg Gruenwald, and PDR staff, eds. 2004. *PDR for Herbal Medicines*. 3rd ed. Atlanta, GA: Thomson Healthcare.

Merchant, R. E., and C. A. Andre. 2001. A review of recent clinical trials of the nutritional supplement *Chlorella pyrenoidosa* in the treatment of fibromyalgia, hypertension, and ulcerative colitis. *Alternative Therapies in Health and Medicine* 7(3):79–91.

Mindell, E., and H. Mundis. 2004. *Earl Mindell's New Vitamin Bible: 25th Anniversary Edition*. New York: Warner Books.

Moldofsky, H., P. Scarisbrick, R. England, and H. Smythe. 1975. Musculoskeletal symptoms and non-REM sleep disturbance in patients with "fibrositis syndrome" and healthy subjects. *Psychosomatic Medicine* 37:341.

Monteleone, P., M. Maj, L. Beinat, M. Natale, and D. Kemali. 1992. Blunting by chronic phosphatidylserine administration of the stress-induced activation of the hypothalamo-pituitary-adrenal axis in healthy men. *European Journal of Clinical Pharmacology* 42:385-388.

Morf, S., B. Amann-Vesti, A. Forster, U. K. Franzeck, R. Koppensteiner, D. Uebelhart, and H. Sprott. 2005. Microcirculation abnormalities in patients with fibromyalgia measured by capillary microscopy and laser fluxmetry. *Arthritis Research and Therapy* 7:R209-R216.

Mountz, J. M., L. A. Bradley, J. G. Modell, R. W. Alexander, and M. Triana-Alexander. 1995. Fibromyalgia in women. Abnormalities of regional cerebral blood flow in the thalamus and the caudate nucleus are associated with low pain threshold levels. *Arthritis & Rheumatism* 38(7):926-938.

Murphy, B. E., F. V. Abbott, C. M. Allison, C. Watts, and A. M. Ghadirian. 2004. Elevated levels of some neuroactive progesterone metabolites, particularly isopregnanolone, in women with chronic fatigue syndrome. *Psychoneuroendocrinology* 29(2):245-268.

Naschitz, J. E., M. Rozenbaum, M. C. Field, S. Enis, H. Manor, D. Dreyfuss, S. Peck, E. R. Peck, J. P. Babich, E. P. Mintz, E. Sabo, G. Slobodin, and I. Rosner. 2005. Cardiovascular reactivity in CFS: Evidence for pathogenic heterogeneity. *Journal of Rheumatology* 32(2):335-339.

Nasralla, M., J. Haier, and G. L. Nicolson. 1999. Multiple mycoplasmal infections detected in blood of patients with chronic fatigue syndrome and/or fibromyalgia syndrome. *European Journal of Clinical Microbiological Infectious Diseases* 18:859-865.

National CFIDS Foundation. 2006. Potential animal (zoonotic) virus identified in patients with chronic fatigue syndrome, multiple sclerosis, and epilepsy. http://www.ncf-net.org/pdf/PressRelease.pdf (accessed July 5, 2006).

NIH (National Institutes of Health). 1998. NIH Consensus Conference. Acupuncture. *Journal of the American Medical Association* 280(17):1518-1524.

NIH (National Institutes of Health) Office of Dietary Supplements. 2004. Dietary supplement fact sheet: Selenium. http://ods.od.nih.gov/factsheets/selenium.asp (accessed January 27, 2007).

——— 2005. Dietary supplement fact sheet: Vitamin D. http://ods.od.nih.gov/factsheets/vitamind.asp (accessed January 27, 2007).

Nijs, J., B. Van de Velde, and K. De Meirleir. 2005. Pain in patients with chronic fatigue syndrome: Does nitric oxide trigger central sensitisation? *Medical Hypotheses* 64(3):558-562.

O'Connell, P., X. Wang, M. Leon-Ponte, C. Griffiths, S. C. Pingle, and G. P. Ahern. 2006. A novel form of immune signaling revealed by transmission of the inflammatory mediator serotonin between dendritic cells and T cells. *Blood* 107(3):1010-1017.

Paiva, E. S., A. Deodhar, K. D. Jones, and R. M. Bennett. 2002. Impaired growth hormone secretion in fibromyalgia patients: Evidence for augmented hypothalamic somatostatin tone. *Arthritis & Rheumatism* 48(1):277-278.

Panerai, A. E., J. Vecchiet, P. Panzeri, P. Meroni, S. Scarone, E. Pizzigallo, M. A. Giamberardino, and P. Sacerdote. 2002. Peripheral blood mononuclear cell beta-endorphin concentration is decreased in chronic fatigue syndrome and fibromyalgia but not in depression: Preliminary report. *Clinical Journal of Pain* 18(4):270-273.

Papaioannou, R., and C. C. Pfeiffer. 1984. Sulfite sensitivity—unrecognized threat. Is molybdenum deficiency the cause? *Journal of Orthomolecular Psychiatry* 13:105-110.

Park, J. H., P. Phothimat, C. T. Oates, M. Hernanz-Schulman, and N. J. Olsen. 1998. Use of P-31 magnetic resonance spectroscopy to detect metabolic abnormalities in muscles of patients with fibromyalgia. *Arthritis & Rheumatism* 41(3):406-413.

PC (Phosphatidylcholine) monograph. 2002. *Alternative Medicine Review* 7(2):150-154.

Pellegrino, M. J., D. Van Fossen, C. Gordon, J. M. Ryan, and G. W. Waylonis. 1989. Prevalence of mitral valve prolapse in primary fibromyalgia: A pilot investigation. *Archives of Physical Medicine and Rehabilitation* 70(7):541-543.

Pierrynowski, M. R., P. M. Tiidus, and V. Galea. 2005. Women with fibromyalgia walk with an altered muscle synergy. *Gait and Posture* 22(3):210-218.

Pimentel, M., E. Chow, and H. Lin. 2000. Eradication of small intestinal bacterial overgrowth reduces symptoms of irritable bowel syndrome. *American Journal of Gastroenterology* 95(12):3503-3506.

Pizzorno, J., and M. Murray. 2006. *Textbook of Natural Medicine.* 3rd ed. St. Louis, MO: Churchill Livingstone Elsevier.

Plioplys, A. V., and S. Plioplys. 1997. Amantadine and L-carnitine treatment of chronic fatigue syndrome. *Neuropsychobiology* 35(1):16-23.

Plotnikoff, G. A., and J. M. Quigley. 2003. Prevalence of severe hypovitaminosis D in patients with persistent, nonspecific musculoskeletal pain. *Mayo Clinic Proceedings* 78(12):1463-1470.

Podell, R. 2003. Reversing eight vicious cycles that block fibromyalgia and chronic fatigue syndrome healing. ImmuneSupport.com (April 29). http://www.immunesupport.com/library/showarticle .cfm/ID/4563 (accessed July 3, 2006).

Puri, B. K. 2004. The use of eicosapentaenoic acid in the treatment of chronic fatigue syndrome. *Prostaglandins Leukotrienes and Essential Fatty Acids* 70(4):399-401.

Rae, C., A. L. Digney, S. R. McEwan, and T. C. Bates. 2003. Oral creatine monohydrate supplementation improves brain performance: A double-blind, placebo-controlled, cross-over trial. *Proceedings of the Royal Society B: Biological Sciences* 270(1529):2147–2150.

Raphael, K. G., M. N. Janal, S. Nayak, J. E. Schwartz, and R. M. Gallagher. 2004. Familial aggregation of depression in fibromyalgia: A community-based test of alternate hypotheses. *Pain* 110(1-2):449-460.

Regland, B., M. Andersson, L. Abrahamsson, J. Bagby, L. E. Dyrehag, and C. G. Gottfries. 1997. Increased concentrations of homocysteine in the cerebrospinal fluid in patients with fibromyalgia and chronic fatigue syndrome. *Scandinavian Journal of Rheumatology* 26(4):301-307.

Reinhard, P., F. Schweinsberg, D. Wernet, and I. Kotter. 1998. Selenium status in fibromyalgia. *Toxicology Letters* 96-97:177-180.

Ringel, Y., A. D. Sperber, and D. A. Drossman. 2001. Irritable bowel syndrome. *Annual Review of Medicine* 52:319-338.

Robertson, M. J., R. S. Schacterle, G. A. Mackin, S. N. Wilson, K. L. Bloomingdale, J. Ritz, and A. L. Komaroff. 2005. Lymphocyte subset differences in patients with chronic fatigue syndrome, multiple sclerosis, and major depression. *Clinical and Experimental Immunology* 141(2):326-332.

Rogers, S. A. 1990. Zinc deficiency as a model for developing chemical sensitivity. *International Clinical Nutrition Review* 10(1):253-258.

Russell, I. 1998. Neurochemical pathogenesis of fibromyalgia. *Zeitschrift für Rheumatologie* 57(Suppl. 2):63-66.

Russell, I. J., J. E. Michalek, J. D. Flechas, and G. E. Abraham. 1995. Treatment of fibromyalgia syndrome with Super Malic: A randomized, double blind, placebo controlled, crossover pilot study. *Journal of Rheumatology* 22:953-958.

Schedel, J. M., H. Tanaka, A. Kiyonaga, M. Shindo, and Y. Schutz. 2000. Acute creatine loading enhances human growth hormone secretion. *Journal of Sports Medicine and Physical Fitness* 40(4):336-342.

Schmitt, W. 2005. Assessing citric acid cycle function. *The Uplink* 35:1. http://www.theuplink.com/TheUplink%20Archives/Forms/News letters%20%20in%20order.aspx (accessed July 8, 2006).

Schore, A. 1999. *Affect Regulation and the Origin of the Self: The Neurobiology of Emotional Development*. Mahwah, NJ: Lawrence Erlbaum Associates.

Scott, L. V., F. Salahuddin, J. Cooney, F. Svec, and T. G. Dinan. 1999. Differences in adrenal steroid profile in chronic fatigue syndrome, in depression and in health. *Journal of Affective Disorders* 54(1-2):129-137.

Scott, L. V., F. Svec, and T. Dinan. 2000. A preliminary study of dehydroepiandrosterone response to low-dose ACTH in chronic fatigue syndrome and in healthy subjects. *Psychiatry Research* 97(1):21-28.

Scott, L. V., J. Teh, R. Reznek, A. Martin, A. Sohaib, and T. G. Dinan. 1999. Small adrenal glands in chronic fatigue syndrome: A preliminary computer tomography study. *Psychoneuroendocrinology* 24(7):759-768.

Sehnert, K. W., and A. C. Croft. 1996. Basal metabolic temperature vs. laboratory assessment in "posttraumatic hypothyroidism." *Journal of Manipulative and Physiological Therapeutics* 19(1):6-12.

Shang, A., K. Huwiler-Muntener, L. Nartey, P. Juni, S. Dorig, J. Sterne, D. Pewsner, and M. Egger. 2005. Are the clinical effects of homoeopathy placebo effects? Comparative study of placebo-controlled trials of homoeopathy and allopathy. *Lancet* 366(9487):726-732.

Shanklin, D. R., M. V. Stevens, M. F. Hall, and D. L. Smalley. 2000. Environmental immunogens and T-cell-mediated responses in fibromyalgia: Evidence for immune dysregulation and determinants of granuloma formation. *Experimental and Molecular Pathology* 69(2):102-118.

Sharma, D. C., and R. Mathur. 1995. Correction of anemia and iron deficiency in vegetarians by administration of ascorbic acid. *Indian Journal of Physiology and Pharmacology* 39:403-406.

Sieverling, C. 2005. The heart of the matter: CFS and cardiac issues. *Newsletter of the CFS and FM support group of Dallas Fort Worth* 7(2, 3). http://www.dfwcfids.org/archive/cfsapr05.pdf (accessed July 8, 2006).

Simons, D., J. Travell, L. Simons, and B. Cummings. 1999. *Myofascial Pain and Dysfunction: The Trigger Point Manual.* 2 volume set. Philadelphia: Lippincott, Williams & Wilkins.

Singh, B., W. Wu, S. Hwang, R. Khorsan, C. Der-Martirosian, S. Vinjamury, C. Wang, and S. Lin. 2006. Effectiveness of acupuncture in the treatment of fibromyalgia. *Alternative Therapies in Health and Medicine* 12(2):34-41.

Smith, A. R., S. V. Shenvi, M. Widlansky, J. H. Suh, and T. M. Hagen. 2004. Lipoic acid as a potential therapy for chronic diseases associated with oxidative stress. *Current Medicinal Chemistry* 11(9):1135-1146.

Smith, J. D., C. M. Terpening, S. O. Schmidt, and J. G. Gums. 2001. Relief of fibromyalgia symptoms following discontinuation of dietary excitotoxins. *Annals of Pharmacotherapy* 35(6):702-706.

Song, G. H., P. H. Leng, K. A. Gwee, S. M. Moochhala, and K. Y. Ho. 2005. Melatonin improves abdominal pain in irritable bowel syndrome patients who have sleep disturbances: A randomised, double blind, placebo controlled study. *Gut* 54(10):1402-1407.

St. Amand, P., and C. C. Marek, 2003. *What Your Doctor May Not Tell You About Fibromyalgia.* Clayton, Victoria: Warner Books.

Staud, R. 2004. Predictors of clinical pain intensity in patients with fibromyalgia syndrome. *Current Rheumatology Reports* 6(4):281-286.

Steinberg, C. 1942. The tocopherols (vitamin E) in the treatment of primary fibrositis. *Journal of Bone and Joint Surgery* 24:411-423.

Suhadolnik, R. J., D. L. Peterson, K. O'Brien, P. R. Cheney, C. V. Herst, N. L. Reichenbach, N. Kon, S. E. Horvath, K. T. Iacono, M. E. Adelson, K. De Meirleir, P. De Becker, R. Charubala, and W. Pfleiderer. 1997. Biochemical evidence for a novel low molecular weight 2-5A-dependent RNase L in chronic fatigue syndrome. *Journal of Interferon and Cytokine Research* 17(7):377-385.

Sullivan, K. 2004. *Naked at Noon.* North Bergen, NJ: Basic Health Publications.

Swezey, R. L., and J. Adams. 1999. Fibromyalgia: A risk factor for osteoporosis. *Journal of Rheumatology* 26(12):2642-2644.

Szelenyi, J. 2001. Cytokines and the central nervous system. *Brain Research Bulletin* 54(4):329-338.

Tarnopolsky, M. A., B. D. Roy, and J. R. MacDonald. 1997. A randomized, controlled trial of creatine monohydrate in patients with mitochondrial cytopathies. *Muscle and Nerve* 20(12):1502-1509.

Tavoni, A., C. Vitali, S. Bombardieri, and G. Pasero. 1987. Evaluation of S-adenosylmethionine in primary fibromyalgia. A double-blind crossover study. *American Journal of Medicine* 83(5A):107-110.

Thiel, R. J. 1998. Natural interventions for people with fibromyalgia. *American Naturopathic Medical Association Monitor* 2(3):5-9. http://www.healthresearch.com/fibro.htm (accessed July 7, 2006).

Thomas, M., and A. Smith. 2005. Primary healthcare provision and chronic fatigue syndrome: A survey of patients' and general practitioners' beliefs. *BMC Family Practice* 6:49. http://www.biomed central.com/content/pdf/1471-2296-6-49.pdf (accessed April 28, 2006).

Van Konynenburg, R. A. 2004. Is glutathione depletion an important part of the pathogenesis of chronic fatigue syndrome? Paper presented at the AACFS Seventh International Conference, Madison, WI, October 8-10. http://www.cfsresearch.org/cfs/research/treatment /15.pdf (accessed July 10, 2006).

Vermeulen, R. C., and H. R. Scholte. 2004. Exploratory open label, randomized study of acetyl- and propionylcarnitine in chronic fatigue syndrome. *Psychosomatic Medicine* 66(2):276-282.

Vernon, S. D., and W. C. Reeves. 2005. Evaluation of autoantibodies to common and neuronal cell antigens in chronic fatigue syndrome. *Journal of Autoimmune Diseases* 2(1):5.

Vinson, J. A., and P. Bose. 1988. Comparative bioavailability to humans of ascorbic acid alone or in a citrus extract. *American Journal of Clinical Nutrition* 48:601-604.

Volkmann, H., J. Norregaard, S. Jacobsen, B. Danneskiold-Samsoe, G. Knoke, and D. Nehrdich. 1997. Double-blind, placebo-controlled cross-over study of intravenous S-adenosyl-L-methionine in patients with fibromyalgia. *Scandinavian Journal of Rheumatology* 26(3):206-211.

Walker, E. A., D. Keegan, G. Gardner, M. Sullivan, D. Bernstein, and W. J. Katon. 1997. Psychosocial factors in fibromyalgia compared with rheumatoid arthritis: II. Sexual, physical, and emotional abuse and neglect. *Psychosomatic Medicine* 59:572-577.

Wallace, D. J., M. Linker-Israeli, D. Hallegua, S. Silverman, D. Silver, and M. H. Weisman. 2001. Cytokines play an aetiopathogenetic role in fibromyalgia: A hypothesis and pilot study. *Rheumatology* 40:743.

Warren, G., M. McKendrick, and M. Peet. 1999. The role of essential fatty acids in chronic fatigue syndrome. A case-controlled study of red-cell membrane essential fatty acids (EFA) and a placebo-controlled treatment study with high dose of EFA. *Acta Neurologica Scandinavica* 99:112-116.

Weissbecker, I., A. Floyd, E. Dedert, P. Salmon, and S. Sephton. 2006. Childhood trauma and diurnal cortisol disruption in fibromyalgia syndrome. *Psychoneuroendocrinology* 31(3):312-324.

Werbach, M. R. 2000. Nutritional strategies for treating chronic fatigue syndrome. *Alternative Medicine Review* 5(2):93-108.

Wheatland, R. 2005. Chronic ACTH autoantibodies are a significant pathological factor in the disruption of the hypothalamic–pituitary–adrenal axis in chronic fatigue syndrome, anorexia nervosa and major depression. *Medical Hypotheses* 65(2):287-295.

Wolfe, F., H. Smythe, M. Yunus, R. Bennett, C. Bombardier, D. Goldenberg, P. Tugwell, S. Campbell, M. Abeles, P. Clark, et al. 1990. The American College of Rheumatology 1990 criteria for the classification of fibromyalgia. Report of the Multicenter Criteria Committee. *Arthritis & Rheumatism* 33(2):160-172.

Yunus, M. B. 2001. Central sensitivity syndromes: A unified concept for fibromyalgia and other similar maladies. *Journal of the Indian Rheumatism Association* 8(1):27-33.

Yunus, M. B., and J. C. Aldag. 1996. Restless legs syndrome and leg cramps in fibromyalgia syndrome: A controlled study. *British Medical Journal* 312:1339.

Zar, S., M. J. Benson, and D. Kumar. 2005. Food-specific serum IgG4 and IgE titers to common food antigens in irritable bowel syndrome. *American Journal of Gastroenterology* 100(7):1550-1557.

Zautra, A. J., R. Fasman, J. W. Reich, P. Harakas, L. M. Johnson, M. E. Olmsted, and M. C. Davis. 2005. Fibromyalgia: Evidence for deficits in positive affect regulation. *Psychosomatic Medicine* 67(1):147-155.

Ziegler, D., H. Nowak, P. Kempler, P. Vargha, and P. A. Low. 2004. Treatment of symptomatic diabetic polyneuropathy with the antioxidant alpha-lipoic acid: A meta-analysis. *Diabetic Medicine* 21(2):114-121.

Lynette Bassman, Ph.D., is associate professor of psychology, specializing in health psychology, at the California School of Professional Psychology of Alliant International University in Fresno, CA. She is the editor of *The Whole Mind: The Definitive Guide to Complementary Treatments for Mind, Mood and Emotions.* Bassman is a survivor of chronic fatigue syndrome; she used alternative medicine approaches for her recovery.

Foreword writer **C. Norman Shealy,** MD, Ph.D., is one of the world's leading experts in pain management. He was among the first physicians ever to specialize in the resolution of chronic pain. A pioneer in developing safe and effective treatments such as Biogenics®, he founded, in 1971, the first comprehensive pain and stress management facility in the country, The Shealy Institute, respected world-wide for its innovative and successful rehabilitation approaches. Over the years, Dr. Shealy's intensive pain and stress management research has resulted in numerous pioneering treatments. His published works total over 275. His seminars and workshops are given worldwide and attended by physicians and lay persons alike. He has acted as consultant to leaders in every specialty, including the personal physicians of Presidents Kennedy and Eisenhower.

more **real tools** for coping with FMS and CFS
from new**harbinger**publications

LIVING BEYOND YOUR PAIN
Using Acceptance & Commitment Therapy to Ease Chronic Pain

$19.95 • Item Code: 4097

THE TRIGGER POINT THERAPY WORKBOOK, SECOND EDITION
Your Self-Treatment Guide for Pain Relief

$19.95 • Item Code: 3759

10 SIMPLE SOLUTIONS TO CHRONIC PAIN
How to Stop Pain from Controlling Your Life

$12.95 • Item Code: 4825

FIBROMYALGIA & CHRONIC FATIGUE SYNDROME
7 Proven Steps to Less Pain & More Energy

$14.95 • Item Code: 4593

FIBROMYALGIA & CHRONIC MYOFASCIAL PAIN, SECOND EDITION
A Survival Manual

$19.95 • Item Code: 2388

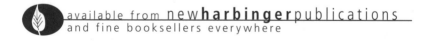